A MOTHER'S LOVE

A MOTHER'S LOVE

Barbara Greene & Vanessa Howard

Quercus

First published in Great Britain in 2011 by

Quercus
21 Bloomsbury Square
London
WC1A 2NS

A CIP catalogue record for this book is available
from the British Library

ISBN 978 1 84916 998 1

10 9 8 7 6 5 4 3 2 1

Printed and bound in Great Britain by
Clays Ltd, St Ives plc

Prologue

In this life, we may learn that little is certain, that happiness can arrive when least expected, or that it is often only recognised in its passing. Live long enough and we learn that it is often the smallest moments that become the most cherished: the moment when a child seeks out a mother's hand to place in its own, or just the sound of the child's sudden laughter from another room.

Life teaches us many things, but perhaps the hardest lesson of all is that with life comes the possibility of death.

From the moment a child is placed in its mother's arms there arrives with it an immediate and permanent acceptance that this new life takes precedence over everything, that it will be supported and nurtured, no matter what the circumstance, the consequence or the sacrifice.

This is of course expected. It is the natural order of things, the very essence of motherhood, and the natural contract between any new mother and her newborn child. It is always in this context that the death of a child – any child – must be understood. There can be no greater tragedy than the death of a child because nothing is so 'unnatural'. Even if that child has reached adulthood, to the mother age simply makes no difference – this grown young man or woman is still and always their child, and their grief is always defined by this unique bond that refuses to be influenced by change or time.

The circumstances of a child's death might be foreseen or unexpected, inevitable or inexplicable, but in every case it is the loss itself that can inhabit every moment of a mother's life, permeate it with the self-flagellating question 'Why do I live when they do not?'

In some instances, however, the events leading up to that loss are of such a nature that they have a particular bearing on the human desolation that inevitably follows. The circumstances of some deaths are so agonising, so difficult to hear or read about, that details leave the listener or the reader numb and overwhelmed with sympathy.

But what if the mother, understanding the precise consequences of her involvement, has knowingly played an 'active' part in that death?

It would be easy, and understandable, to recoil from such a fact, to question how such a thing could be possible, or glibly to suggest that the mother had no choice, but how are we really to understand an act that appears to go so much against human nature and nurture?

In an attempt to answer these difficult and imponderable questions, among other stories recounted in this book we examine and analyse the circumstances and actions of two mothers, Kay Gilderdale and Frances Inglis. Within days of each other, these two women, both in their fifties, suddenly entered the public spotlight, each standing trial in front of a British judge and jury accused of crimes connected with the deaths of their children – thirty-one-year-old Lynn Gilderdale and twenty-two-year-old Tom Inglis.

As with every death, each had its own narrative, its own singular moments of private tragedy; but the two cases differed greatly in detail, both in the events leading up to each death and in the circumstances of the deaths themselves.

The end for Kay Gilderdale's daughter Lynn came after a lengthy struggle with an illness which had struck early in her teens, robbed her of life's joys, and resulted in her mother devotedly caring for her every hour of the day from then on. Frances Inglis's son Tom suffered no such drawn-out torment but, in a terrible turn of fate, fell victim to a tragic late-night accident that instantly transformed him from a healthy young man to a hospitalised victim, unable to care for himself, eat, or even breathe unaided.

What these two grim cases do have in common, however, is that both mothers faced a choice: to allow their children to continue existing in the cruel condition that had befallen them – or to do something about it. And it was the choice that each of them made that led to their respective trials and placed them at the centre of the controversial debates that ensued as press and public argued the rights and wrongs of their actions – and the law's view of their deeds.

One thing that was not challenged either by the courts or public opinion was the motive behind the actions of the mothers involved: that they were driven to act by their deep love for their children was universally agreed.

But that love led Kay Gilderdale and Frances Inglis (Frankie to her family) to become the focus of a whole range of questions from a society that was, and remains, increasingly concerned about the medicalisation of death.

Each of us will know, or will come to know, an elderly family member or friend wracked by illness but sustained beyond consciousness, technically alive through the intervention of drugs and mechanical apparatus, but a physical and mental husk of the person they once were.

Is this delayed, protracted and obstructed process of death what we would wish for ourselves or tolerate for those we love were an alternative and humane route available? In so many other aspects of our lives we expect our views to be taken into account, to be respected; we expect choice, and yet in this most crucial aspect of life – our deaths – the law is unequivocal. Life is to be sustained, no matter how poor its 'quality'.

And so we have reached a point where medical efficiency outstrips human will. There is a grey area within which doctors are expected to function – a blurred world which demands that the law must be obeyed in the face of the clear futility of maintaining a life that functions only at a mechanical level.

The apparatus exists to keep lungs moving like a bellows, to keep a depleted body fed thorough a gastric tube, but eventually families begin to say 'enough'. It is then, perhaps, that 'do not resuscitate' signs are posted at the bedside or the request for the withdrawal of water and nutrition is made and the patient is effectively starved to death.

Is this what we imagined death to be?

At this crossroads of medical advances and individual rights we have, inevitably perhaps, become accustomed, or even immune, to hearing and reading certain stock phrases that have entered everyday language: 'mercy killing', 'assisted suicide', 'assisted death', 'suicide tourism' and so on.

And although every example is unique, these phrases and the complex issues behind them came to haunt Kay Gilderdale and Frances Inglis, two mothers already struggling with unimaginable grief.

As well as examining in detail what happened to the Gilderdale and Inglis families before, during and after their trials, we look also at the decisions that others took when faced with the life-and-death dilemma of their loved ones' plight.

The legal position, too, is evaluated here. Its guidelines are constantly being reviewed in response not only to public pressure, but also to the detailed and articulate concern expressed by high-profile public figures, church leaders, lawyers, doctors, and pressure groups on both sides of the argument. Also, the feelings of those most closely affected by events; the fathers, sons, daughters, lovers and friends are taken into account.

But, above all, it is the anguish of the mothers, those women whose love faced the greatest test of all, which is the focus of what follows. What they and their families endured was harrowing, and triggered by simple misfortune; a sudden illness in one case, an unforeseen accident in the other.

With tens of thousands of road traffic accidents each year and thousands more admitted to hospitals with sudden illness, no family is immune to the possibility of a loved one suffering a similar fate to those described here. We know that tragedy could face each and every one of us and it leaves us all to confront the unthinkable question: What would *I* do and would it be right?

1

Everything to Live For

It would be hard to find a less dramatic setting for a story of unrelieved heartbreak than the village of Stonegate.

Hidden in the East Sussex countryside, its nearest main route for traffic, a few minutes' drive away along a country lane, isn't even an 'A' road; it's the virtually anonymous B2099 between Wadhurst and Ticehurst to the north. Even Stonegate's station, on the main line between London and Hastings, isn't in the 'centre' of the village but lies, isolated, a mile to the south, overlooking the Rother Valley.

Stonegate grew at the junction of two Roman roads, and one can't avoid the thought that perhaps there was more hustle and bustle two thousand years ago than there is nowadays. Quiet as it is, Stonegate is not a picture-postcard village, it is not of the half-timbered pub–duck pond–cricket-on-the-green variety so beloved of tourist board brochures. It is too nondescript for such imagery and, in that respect, far more familiar.

Tucked away from sight in a quiet cul-de-sac in this sleepy part of the country is a sprinkling of post-war bungalows; the type of homes that are synonymous with those seeking peace and quiet in which to live unfussy and tranquil lives. Neat gardens with cropped lawns, trellises standing to attention alongside the front doors, ample space in the driveways for two cars or more – the sort of houses in the kind of village that is classically described as a place where 'nothing happens'. Not usually, anyway. But in one corner of that road leading nowhere, a tragedy was unfolding.

In the back bedroom of one of these houses, behind curtains permanently drawn to keep the sunlight away from ultra-sensitive eyes, a young, pale-faced woman was lying in bed. Surrounded by photos and ornaments, she lay on a sheepskin in an effort to prevent her getting bedsores. Her head rested on a folded towel because her neck had become too weak to hold it up. A tube, through which liquid food passed in order to sustain her, entered through her nose, and another intravenous line sent drugs straight into her chest. She had no feeling in her legs, although the bones were at risk of fracture should she be moved too quickly, and since the sixth month of her illness, whenever she attempted to sit up she would lose consciousness.

Once, this young woman had been a vibrant teenager. Now she could neither swallow nor speak. Despite every effort made to provide her with every comfort, nothing could bring respite from her intolerable and never-ending pain.

And there, always by her side and caring for her constantly, was her mother. A mother whose love for her daughter could – and would – never be doubted And whose devotion was remarkable, even by the standards of that strongest of bonds – a mother's love for her child.

Yet this was a woman whose actions would spark a national debate and who would find herself in the dock not only of the Crown Court but in the far tougher arena of public opinion. Because, as she ran from her daughter's room it was to find tablets that she could crush up and give to her. Later she would call Exit, the euthanasia information line, and wonder why, with the morphine her daughter now had in her system, was she still alive?

In the weeks and months to come, those who heard about the case would ask, how could she? Yet all would come to wonder what they too might be capable of.

Nothing about Kay Gilderdale can be understood without understanding her daughter Lynn, a truly remarkable person on so many levels. Lynn had once been an ordinary girl, which is not to say that she was without her talents, far from it. She had excelled at a good many things. As well as learning to sail a dinghy by herself, she played the piano and the clarinet, had won ballet prizes by the age of nine, and at ten captained the netball team. Bright and always on the move, she loved swimming, cycling and dancing.

By the time she was fourteen, Lynette Gilderdale, who had always been called Lynn, was a lively, fun-loving girl with a busy social life. She could be headstrong but her parents ensured that she was respectful towards others and they took a quiet pride in the way their youngest child relished life. Kay would always look up at the clock just before she expected to hear her daughter run into the house, bursting to tell her about her day.

The early teens are a taxing time for parents. Lynn's father, Richard, was a police sergeant and so knew more than most the risks that come when children are gaining their independence. It is a difficult balancing act between wanting your child to enjoy more freedoms and recognising that the ability to form good judgement only comes with experience. And the wish to keep them close and safe from harm never diminishes.

Parents want their children to take gradual and steady steps towards adulthood when, in reality, adolescents more often tend to take clumsy leaps. Perhaps that has always been the way of things, and no doubt most parents once got into scrapes of their own, which is a necessary part of growing up. Parents push away their most dread thoughts and reassure themselves with the knowledge that, whatever mishap befalls their child, they will always be on hand to pick up the pieces and dry the tears.

In 1991, with Bryan Adams's 'Everything I Do (I Do It For You)' dominating the charts and *The Silence of the*

Lambs cleaning up at the Oscars, Lynn turned fourteen. She was popular and had a wide circle of friends, and was naturally pushing for greater freedoms. Her parents were happy that she enjoyed going to the youth centre with her friends, but they were also relieved that she still liked to spend time with them and her elder brother, Steve. She still welcomed being together as a family.

In November that year, Lynn's class was informed her year would receive the BCG vaccine. As well as being a welcome distraction from the usual lesson plan, it was something to giggle about as pupils lined up to see the nurse. The vaccine was used to prevent TB (tuberculosis), a disease that still proves devastating in many parts of the world but which has been contained in the UK for some time thanks to better sanitation and the once routine immunisation of children at the age of thirteen. Success has been such that, since 2005, the vaccine has been phased out and is only given to those children thought to be at a high risk of contracting the disease.

A little while after the vaccination at school, Lynn began to feel unwell, as if she were getting a cold. Vaccinations do trouble some children but Lynn's health had always been robust and it didn't seem to be anything to worry about.

Mothers can't help but monitor even minor coughs and colds with a wary eye. GPs and health visitors reassure new mothers that they should be thankful for every common ailment as each time a child battles a virus a profile of its characteristics is stored away. These profiles act as building blocks for the immune system, allowing it to mature and to quickly produce antibodies should the virus ever appear again.

This is the type of information and advice mothers call on when sitting up at night struggling to lower a child's fever, trusting that it will pass, believing that with today's medical practices, nothing seriously amiss can happen. Ailments can be caught, treated and cured; even those that only a few generations ago led to child mortalities.

Lynn seemed to rally during the night after her inoculation, and decided that she was well enough to go back to school the next day. But she was sent home. And then she was sent home again . . . and again . . .

And then, she never went back.

The next few weeks and months were like nothing Kay had ever experienced. Lynn developed one illness after another: Influenza, bronchitis, tonsillitis, chest infection, glandular fever. Her system was clearly under attack and just as she seemed to begin shaking off one ailment, another would assail her. Kay, who had trained as an auxiliary nurse, was baffled. Her daughter was certainly 'run down' but this series of infections was new to her; both Steve and Lynn had always rallied after a bug and been themselves within a day or so.

Suddenly, Kay and Richard found themselves taken up with battling whatever illness their daughter was suffering and they began to fear that her problems weren't caused by the 'normal' range of viruses that youngsters get from time to time.

Despite any number of visits to doctors, and countless courses of antibiotics prescribed, Lynn was deteriorating. By February 1992, she was very ill indeed. Her limbs, especially her legs, weakened profoundly, her memory began to suffer, and she endured widespread pain. The top half of her body became floppy and unresponsive, mimicking the signs parents are told to watch for in dangerously ill toddlers, and yet only a few months earlier, this had been a teenage girl in rude health.

It was impossible to reconcile this girl with the one that Kay and Richard knew and loved, the girl who, laughing, raced her brother along the beach. As well as being forced to put up with long periods of pain and discomfort, Lynn was also confused and fearful, asking her parents again and again what was wrong with her.

They could give their daughter no answers. The catalogue of illnesses was growing out of control. Mothers question themselves over and over again, wondering what signs they perhaps missed; was there something they should – or could – have done? Or done differently?

Parents tick through the stages of childhood well aware of terrible illnesses that can beset healthy children at different stages of development; meningitis, childhood leukaemia and even undiagnosed heart conditions that can claim the lives of those who have never been ill.

All parents come to hear of children who succumb to terminal illnesses, all trust and pray that it won't happen to theirs. The biggest concern for Kay and Richard was that there might be an underlying reason for Lynn's collapsing immunity, and that it had not been detected. If Lynn had an underlying serious disease, it had to be found. Then, God willing, a course of treatment could begin.

Set against this fear that something was fundamentally wrong with Lynn was disbelief. It seemed impossible that she would not turn the corner and return to her old self. It had been a dreadful few months but the family hoped that it would all pass; that they would look back in years to come and shake their heads as they remembered 'that awful time'.

In due course they were reassured that Lynn was not suffering from any form of childhood cancer. It was a relief, of course, but the question remained: what was wrong? It was three months before her illness could be diagnosed; the answer, when it came, was worryingly vague. Lynn had ME.

It was then that a new and terrifying nightmare began.

Myalgic Encephalopathy, or ME – originally called Myalgic Encephalomyelitis – is an illness of uncertain cause affecting about 250,000 people in Britain alone. It is grouped with certain other conditions: Chronic Fatigue Syndrome

(CFS), Post-Viral Fatigue Syndrome (PVFS) or Chronic Fatigue Immune Dysfunction Syndrome (CFIDS).

Despite confusion over its origin, the illness has no doubt existed as long as any other. It may well be the case, for example, that Victorian references to a condition then known as 'the vapours' was in fact ME. The illness was first noted in medical literature in 1934, but it was not until 1954 that an attempt was made to document it in what became known as the Wallis Description.

Two years later, the former Chief Medical Officer in the UK, Sir Donald Acheson, carried out the first major review of the condition, and from 1962 ME appeared in standard neurological handbooks. It seems incredible that after almost fifty years the illness remains seriously misunderstood – and not just by the public. Far more worryingly, it is not understood, and sometimes not accepted, by a number of medical practitioners.

In the 1980s, references to the illness began to appear in the media. Many felt that ME wasn't really an illness, but something 'all in the mind', co-opted by people who somehow or other struggled to cope with the strain of living in a competitive and high-paced society. It was around this time that it gained its pejorative term, 'yuppie flu'. The misconceptions wrapped around the illness led some to take a dangerously dismissive attitude, and this would impact on Lynn, her family, and the thousands of others who have contracted the condition.

Anybody can be affected by ME, no matter their background, age, social status or previous health record. The disease results in a systemic dysfunction of the central nervous system. Treatment consists of trying to contain a range of chronic symptoms, but there is no clear understanding of how, in numerous cases, to prevent the disease from shutting down the body's homeostasis – the brain's ability to regulate vital functions.

Severe and debilitating fatigue, painful muscles and joints, disordered sleep, gastric disturbances, and poor memory and concentration are commonplace symptoms. For some, the condition is far more extreme, effectively shutting down the nerve centres that control cardiovascular, hormonal, sensory, digestive, cognitive, visual and spinal nerve tract functions.

In many cases, the onset of ME is believed to be triggered by a virus and is linked to a viral infection. Other triggers can include the aftermath of an operation or an accident, although some people experience a slow, insidious development seemingly not linked to any one event.

Around a quarter of those who contract the illness go on to develop serious and ongoing complications. To date, there is no known cure and no universally effective treatment. Treatments that have reduced particular symptoms in some have proved ineffective or counter-productive in others.

Predisposing factors to developing ME are thought to include having other sufferers in the family; altered immune response possibly linked to previous infections such as glandular fever or hepatitis; exhaustion and mental stress from, for example, athletic over-training, or work-related stress.

Results from studies indicate that ME often becomes a chronic and very disabling illness, with full recovery occurring in only a minority of cases. And, most telling, some of the most serious cases are said to involve teenagers aged between thirteen and sixteen – Lynn Gilderdale's age group.

The Gilderdale family, who knew nothing of this, soon found themselves trapped in a spiral of fear, anxiety, and medical mismanagement of their daughter's illness.

'Give it a little longer', the family were advised, the belief being that it was inconceivable that such an athletic and outgoing girl could be diminished by infection for long. Lynn began to have difficulty walking, and soon the medical advice insisted that she should adopt a regime of rest followed by structured if gentle exercise.

It was a fraught situation for Kay. Lynn was weak in a way that she had never seen her before; she struggled to stand, let alone join her mother on a walk around the village. The urge to get an ill child back on its feet, both literally and metaphorically, is a strong one; it is only natural to want to see the worst behind you and a return to normality, but Kay sensed that Lynn needed continued rest. Nevertheless, she was told that a routine combining exercise with rest was the most natural way for a body to regain its strength. This was accepted wisdom and certainly seemed rational in many respects, but watching her daughter struggle to put one foot in front of the other was heartbreaking. What on earth was happening to Lynn . . .?

By May, the girl's health had plummeted to a new low. She was reduced to using a wheelchair and, as summer came, her voice began to fail. The voice that had filled the house, the sound of the laughter Kay used to hear as Stephen and Lynn chased each other around the garden, was reduced to a whisper.

But worse was to come: soon Lynn began to have difficulty swallowing, and it was suggested that if the illness continued in this form, she would have to be fed through a tube. Sitting with her daughter hour after hour, Kay worried about what lay ahead. Her escalating anxiety would turn into terrible fear when Lynn's unresponsive limbs went into bouts of violent spasm that only ceased when Lynn fell unconscious.

The physical impact of the illness was staggering, but even harder to witness and to bear was Lynn's cognitive decline. When Kay walked into Lynn's room, her daughter seemed to struggle to recognise her.

Perhaps it was no more than exhaustion, but on one occasion when Richard was wheeling her to the car, Lynn asked, 'What's a car?' Richard continued to talk to his daughter calmly and placed her gently in the car, then asked her to put on her seatbelt. It broke his heart to realise that she didn't know what he meant. His smart and funny girl, the one who could match him in any verbal bout, the girl whose face would light up when he called her his 'best friend', was lost to more than physical pain and illness. She had been cut adrift and left struggling to coordinate her thoughts and her understanding of the world. Talking to her was like talking to someone lost to dementia, yet this was a girl not yet sixteen years old. It was an intolerable cruelty for Lynn and for her devoted and desperate parents.

Battling to help Lynn manage her pain and distress was difficult enough, but what the Gilderdales found themselves up against in the medical community made matters much harder to bear. Typically, one doctor remarked, 'It's okay, you've got a fashionable disease. It will go away in time.' No doubt the comment was meant to reassure but in fact it exposed a wider unspoken suspicion that a significant aspect of ME was 'all in the mind'.

No doubt such scepticism was reinforced with the return of test after test that showed negative results for serious diseases. Had it been proved that Lynn had leukaemia for example, sympathy would have been automatic and a prescribed course of action taken. However, seeing a teenager lie listlessly in bed without a recognised and understood label attached to her condition, triggered responses in certain medical staff that can only be described as cruelly lacking in any compassion or understanding.

Of course, it can be argued that the doctors and nurses involved had the best of intentions in attempting to force Lynn to 'snap out of it'. All parents know that children have to learn that self-indulgence and 'crying wolf' simply won't wash. For those who work in doctors' surgeries and hospitals, hypochondriacs and attention-seekers are commonplace. There may be underlying psychological reasons why some people constantly need to seek medical attention and sympathy when they are not in fact ill; in many instances it validates a need to receive the comfort that was denied them in childhood, but medical staff come to recognise – and resent – those wasting valuable time and resources might be depriving those with legitimate needs.

In some cases, attention seeking without foundation can be so profound and deep seated, that it is a recognised psychiatric condition known as Munchausen Syndrome, in which the person fakes or induces symptoms of illness.

Naturally, doctors aware of the syndrome test for it accordingly, but imagine the impact this can have on a genuinely very ill and frightened girl. Imagine being told that you are pretending and that you need to grow up and stop being a silly. Imagine being left alone for hours as pain courses through your system, while staff wait to see if you will get out of bed and sort yourself out. Lynn seemed to suffer spasms at the same time of day – could she be staging them for effect, the medics wondered? To find out, the clock was taken from her room and she was lied to about what time it was. Yet the attacks still occurred, as they always had, at the same time of day.

The attempts to discover what could lie at the root of Lynn's alleged 'psychological' problems were even more distressing than those simple tests of physical will: Lynn was quizzed as to whether she was being abused at home. With hindsight, it is easy to be appalled at such treatment being meted out to a frightened and confused teenager, but such were the doubts and ignorance about the symptoms and impact of ME at the time, that it was almost inevitable that other causes of a condition such as Lynn's would be sought.

Munchausen Syndrome is a serious psychiatric disorder. Sufferers either mimic or even create symptoms in order to gain medical attention. It is not unknown for those with the disorder to self harm by, for example, deliberately infecting a cut or injecting themselves with toxic substances in order to mimic serious infections. Documented cases include instances of people undergoing scores of unnecessary medical procedures and hundreds of hospital admissions; leading some to want to rename the condition 'Medical Abuse Syndrome' to underline the impact of the condition on the institutions that deal with them.

A greater concern comes with a variant of the condition known as Munchausen Syndrome by Proxy. Those mentally afflicted with this condition tend to inflict suffering on others, very often children, in order to gain attention. It can be highly dangerous, as in the case of Beverly Allitt, the nurse known as the 'Angel of Death', who injected babies and toddlers in her care in order to drive extreme medical intervention as she watched. Her actions led to the death of four children, and injuries to five others before she was caught and arrested in 1991 – the same year that Lynn Gilderdale first became ill.

With so much publicity surrounding the Allitt case, perhaps it is not surprising that questions were asked about Lynn. After all, Allitt's work colleagues at the children's ward in Grantham had been hoodwinked for months while she was carrying out her attacks.

There were some who wondered if Kay Gilderdale had Munchausen Syndrome and if her daughter had inherited the condition. One of the warning signs of Munchausen in an adult can come when a child in their care presents a series of medical conditions that do not respond to treatment, that are persistent and unexplained. It was unfortunate that Lynn's conditions seemed at first to mirror this pattern. Set against this misunderstanding was a scared child wondering what was happening and parents whose hearts broke because they couldn't tell her.

Kay initially believed hospital was the best place for Lynn to receive care and treatment and to have her ongoing symptoms properly monitored. But over time it became clear that Lynn was not improving, and Kay sensed in her a growing anxiety. By the end of the summer, Lynn could move only her little finger and was being fed through a tube. Kay wanted her home.

The Gilderdales were told that removing her from the ward could prove fatal but Kay no longer felt confident that her daughter was at peace there. The family talked through the practical implications of bringing Lynn home. Kay would have to give up her job in bookkeeping and the strain on her would be considerable, but she did not hesitate; she had always put her children first and would continue to do so.

Once home, mother and daughter quickly established a routine of care that, put simply, consisted in meeting Lynn's needs, sitting with her, and providing her with constant reassurance. Kay made it clear that she had no desire to be anywhere else but at Lynn's side, and that they would fight the disease together no matter how many months, or even years, it might take.

Kay and Lynn soon developed a series of signs, a language that allowed Lynn to communicate with minimal effort. Although Lynn was trapped in a body that was failing, Kay could still recognise the determination her daughter had always shown before her illness. She had always been a resolute character and she and her mother now focused positively on the future, talking together about what they would do when the illness was finally at an end. Gradually, Kay saw some of her daughter's spirit return.

The hardest times were the night times. Lynn needed continual rest but she would wake in terror, recalling some of the helplessness she had felt in hospital. She seemed terrified of doctors and nurses now and it took almost three years for those nightmares to subside.

During the early stages of Lynn's illnesses, Richard and Kay had been concerned about the amount of school time that their daughter was missing. At one point, still believing that she would eventually go back to school, they had arranged for a home tutor (paid for by the Education Authority) to try and make sure that Lynn didn't fall too far behind the rest of her class. The effort had proved too much for Lynn. The sessions exhausted her and she had found it impossible to concentrate, so they had to let the tutor go.

Now that Lynn was at home, Kay wanted other aspects of her daughter's former life to have a part to play in what was hoped would be her eventual recovery. She was delighted that some of Lynn's closest friends still wanted to show how much they cared for her. They would send notes and cards and they would visit, and although Lynn could no longer interact with them as she once had, Kay knew how much the gestures of friendship mattered.

Lynn had always been close to her mother and even though she was often completely overwhelmed with pain and discomfort she never failed to think about others. She worried about her mum: she knew that Kay was sacrificing any life outside the home by committing to caring for her and it worried her. Kay was only thirty-seven years old when she gave up her career to become her daughter's full-time carer and they talked about what this meant. Kay reassured Lynn that this was the only place she could imagine being, that nothing else mattered, not her work nor her social life nor anything outside the family. All mothers will recognise the fundamental truth that what really matters and comes before all else is their child's health and wellbeing.

And, of course, Lynn would surely turn a corner soon . . .

2

'There are things worse than death'

—

Most local news stories never break through to the national papers; if they do, it might be because it is a quiet news day and a story about a bus crash with a fatality or two can work its way up to the third or fourth news item or merit a paragraph in the 'round-up' column.

For those who've lost a loved one, this brief dismissal can add even further to a sense of loss; the page is turned, the world continues regardless. Indeed, all of us will have glanced at an item about a road accident, an overdose, someone falling to their death, a toddler drowning and so on, and with a shake of the head, turned our attention to the next news item.

But in those few seconds of reading, perhaps we sub-consciously consider the question, does this affect me? If it does, if it touches a nerve, a fear that we are each at risk, vulnerable to something that we cannot control, the story will develop and expand. This is what makes the differ-ence from a news editor's perspective, this is what gives a story 'legs'.

Sometimes the story is big from the start and instantly begins to spiral – the report of a missing child for example. Fears about a child being abducted are, on one level, irrational: the risks today are in reality no greater than they ever were, and children are overwhelmingly more at risk in their own homes than from unknown predators.

When Shannon Matthews was reported missing, the story became an overnight countrywide sensation. When it transpired that her mother had been instrumental in her own daughter's 'disappearance', concern turned to anger and outrage, but there was also a measure of relief. At least there was no new Roy Whiting or Ian Huntley at large to threaten the lives of little girls, so readers could forget about the story and move on.

Other stories about the darker side of human nature take longer to occupy the headlines and capture our attention because the pertinence to each of us is not clear at first. Most murder victims, for example, know their attackers, so when we read about a man arrested after his ex-wife is found dead, we rarely register surprise because, consciously or not, we all hold certain preconceived notions about murder. Thus, of the nine hundred or so homicides that occur each year, few will make readers sit up and express dismay.

If a woman is the killer, however, the ground begins to shift.

Female killers disturb our preconceptions, our beliefs and expectations – and if a woman is responsible for the death of her child, the stage is set for a frenzied and detailed examination of what could possibly have led to such a monstrous act.

News agencies are usually the first to break a story, feeding it through to local and national papers – thirty to forty words that light a fuse. In this case, on 24 November 2008, the feed ran 'A mother from Dagenham who was charged with attempting to murder her brain-damaged son will appear in court after he was found dead at a rehabilitation centre.'

The woman would be identified as fifty-six-year-old Frances Inglis, mother of twenty-two-year-old Thomas Inglis. A spokesman for the Neuro Centre in Hertfordshire where Thomas had died said, 'The staff are very upset and are working very hard with the police to establish what happened.'

Slowly, the details began to emerge. Thomas had been involved in a road accident the year before and had originally been placed in a brain injury unit in Essex, nearer to his mother's home in Dagenham. It was some time later that he was transferred to the unit in Sawbridgeworth in Hertfordshire. As the death had occurred in that county, it was a spokeswoman for Hertfordshire Police who issued the simple statement, 'All circumstances surrounding this tragic incident will be investigated.'

Murder investigations operate on two levels. Initially, following an arrest, the procedures are clear and precise:

wheels are set in motion to charge the suspect, who is obliged to appear at a Magistrate's Court where the charge is read out and a plea is entered. Once the police have concluded their investigation, the case file is passed on to the Crown Prosecution Service – the CPS – and the decision is theirs to make as to whether the case will proceed to trial. Many months might pass, but the wheels turn and grind on inexorably until a conclusion is reached, whatever the outcome.

On the other level, those tasked with investigating the circumstances surrounding a sudden death know that what they uncover stands to be far from clear and precise. Each death acts as a still point in a turbulent, obscure, terrifying, and often violent human story. The truth will be hard to establish and, very often, the truth may not even be clear to the perpetrator who initiated the events and is now caught up in their consequences.

Why do people kill? Detectives are loath to answer questions such as this. They emphasise repeatedly that their function is only to establish the facts of what happened and to collect evidence in support of their conclusions. It is not theirs to reason why. And yet motive is fundamental to the equation.

In criminal law, the prosecution has to establish the *mens rea* (Latin for 'guilty mind') as well as the *actus reas* ('guilty act'); this means that the accused must possess not only the physical ability to kill, but also the mental capacity to understand that their actions will lead to the death of the victim. Crudely put, those accused of murder have to pick up the knife and have the intention to kill.

This may seem a blindingly obvious point to make, but it is crucial within the British legal system. British law is, like the British Constitution itself, unique in that it does not rest on a series of rights laid down in a constitution, but has evolved over hundreds of years case by case. It changes subtly, and sometimes substantially, as society changes. Governments, of course, make laws that have a dramatic impact on the legal system – the abolition of capital punishment in 1965, for example – but most law is built on precedent, altering course gradually as judges make new rulings and the sentiments of a changing society are taken into account.

The establishing of *mens rea* and *actus reus* has played a vital part in British justice. If, for example, an acutely mentally incapacitated person dropped a brick that led to a fatality, they would not have been judged suitable to be tried for murder. The interpretation of what it means to have a 'guilty mind' – to want or have the desire to murder – saved many from the gallows before Britain abolished the death penalty.

'Want' is an amorphous but key element in assembling an understanding of what has led to someone's death. British courts differ from the American model in that motive does not have to be established, but is significant in judging *mens rea*. When the police open a file on a murder investigation, consideration of motive will help frame the direction of their enquiry. Detectives may not like to talk ethics but, as one commented, 'Show me how someone lived, and I can show you how they will have died.'

Unpremeditated murder generally arises from anger or jealousy that runs out of control; sexually based killings are sometimes the unintended result of certain activities or – as in the case of Myra Hindley and Ian Brady, or Peter Sutcliffe, to name only a couple of notorious examples – are the expression of serious psychological disorder.

Greed, all too evident week in week out to serious crime units, can be a motive of both unpremeditated and pre-meditated murder – a man mugged and killed for the contents of his wallet, or because he got in the way of a major armed robbery, through to the planned disposing of a family member to gain their fortune.

If greed seeks to kill for gain, rage is a murderous explosion that seeks relief from anger. In trying to establish motive, detectives will ask the victim's friends and family whether they were in conflict with anybody particular, and they will frequently find that the victim knew their killer – a spouse, a partner, an ex-lover. Amidst the denials, the lies and the obfuscation, simple patterns emerge. The impact of violent action rarely, if ever, brings the material or emotional rewards the killer sought.

*

When Hertfordshire police began to look into the nature of Thomas Inglis's death, suspicion fell – not for the first time – on his mother, Frances Inglis. It was clear that all family members would need to be interviewed but, in particular, Frances, around whom a complex picture was already emerging in connection with her son's well-being.

Tom was a pipe-fitter by trade, a happy and lively young man with a wide group of friends and good prospects. His parents, both known to be devoted to their three sons, had been separated for some time but remained on good terms for the sake of their boys. Tom lived close by with his girl-friend but would sometimes stay over with his mother, where he shared a bedroom with one of his brothers.

Frances was studying nursing. She had many years' experience as a community support worker for adults with learning disabilities and felt the time was right to gain pro-fessional qualifications to help and enhance her career. After all, her boys were now adults, each with his own life to live and, like many mothers at this stage, it was impor-tant to think about how to shape the last years of her working life.

Like Tom, Frances knew a good many people and was well liked. She was known to be a good neighbour, and was thought of as one of those women who help make commu-nities function for the good of all. Over the years, the

London Borough of Barking and Dagenham – an area once famous for the Ford car plant and as the birthplace of comedian Dudley Moore and singer Sandie Shaw – has seen many changes, but a close-knit community remained in the suburb of Dagenham itself. Frances was part of that community, and a person who could be relied on to be on hand to help out anyone who might need her.

If asked about her hopes for the future, Frances would have thought first about her boys, wishing to see them happy and settled and starting families of their own; then perhaps she would have thought about her nursing training at London Southbank University, hoping it would go well. Hers would have been the kind of quiet ambitions many of us have, not for great wealth or fame but for the seamless and quiet happiness of those we love.

It is perhaps the random nature of tragedy that makes it so very hard to bear. A single unexpected moment, an ill-thought out impulse, a series of otherwise unremarkable events that end in sudden catastrophe ... How can someone be fine one moment and struck down the next? When a tragic incident occurs, a family, lost in grief, can be left with the cruel echo of that question for years to come.

And, of course, that tragedy comes out of nowhere, transforming in that moment an ordinary family to one redefined by shock, changing its emotional landscape forever. For the Inglis family, that moment came on a typical Friday night, at the end of a working week when

Tom Inglis was meeting a group of friends for a night out in Becontree Heath, near Dagenham. It would mean a few beers of course but where was the harm in that?

By their late teens, most young men want to hang out with friends and enjoy themselves at weekends, but mothers dread the onset of these nights of drinking. Not without reason: it's on these occasions in the pub when young men are most at risk from 'stranger violence', unpremeditated attacks fuelled by alcohol abuse and aggression.

Parents lecture their children about not taking unnecessary risks, about sensible drinking and about the importance of avoiding trouble. Filmed footage from High Streets across the UK have shown 'binge Britain' at its worst, capturing images of girls lying insensible on pavements, and random and brutal acts of violence among groups of drunken young men.

The horror stories of such incidents have dominated the last few years of domestic weekend news coverage – young men being fatally stabbed on a night out as they try to protect a friend from attack; others losing their lives when they were no more than innocent bystanders. When a killer is 'unknown' to his victim, these are the circumstances that make up the rump of those statistics.

Parents are told by their children not to worry, that random acts of violence will not be something that troubles them, nor would they ever get themselves involved in such behaviour. Of course, parents have to allow their young adult children the freedom to find their own way, and anxiety gradually diminishes and disappears if nothing untoward happens over the first months and then the years. Acceptance comes and trust develops: after all, young adults have to learn how to handle themselves and how to avoid trouble.

In his early twenties, Tom Inglis was no novice. He was accustomed to going out and enjoying himself without putting himself in harm's way. He was no troublemaker and, more importantly, he knew how to give any signs of trouble a wide berth. That Friday night began no differently from any other; he should have made his way home in the early hours as he always did, he might have had a hangover to worry about in the morning, but also plenty to report about the fun he had with his friends the night before.

That Friday fell on a summer's night in the first week of July 2007, and the streets were busy. It was shortly after the smoking ban had been introduced, and a number of drinkers found themselves standing outside the Ship & Anchor in order to light up and enjoy a cigarette. By closing time in the early hours of the morning, the street atmosphere was boisterous and noisy as various groups stumbled out of the pub shouting to friends about what venue to call into next or debating whether to call it a night and look for a taxi.

But as the police well know, the late-night cat calls and laughter can so easily flare into jostling and disagreement. Officers on night duty, trained to manage and defuse situations as they crop up, are accustomed to intervening as voices are raised and aggression levels rise – as are security staff working in pubs and clubs. In the main, even those who are highly intoxicated can be persuaded to walk away, but the fault lines are always there, just below the surface; a misheard word, a misjudged punch, and mayhem follows.

That night outside the Ship & Anchor, as a fight in which he was not involved spilled out into the street, Tom Inglis was caught by a blow. It wasn't aimed at him but it split his lip. His friends gathered round and, although the cut wasn't too bad, it was bleeding and looked as though it might need stitches to staunch the blood.

Ambulance crews arrived within minutes of the fight breaking out. Assessments were made and although Tom could technically be classified as 'walking wounded' the paramedics took the view that his cut should be checked over at A&E.

Over any given weekend, some seventy per cent of admissions to accident and emergency units throughout Britain are now thought to be a result of alcohol abuse. A quarter of young men are believed to drink double the daily guidelines at least once a week, particularly at the weekend. The cost to the NHS of these peak-time casualties is close to three billion pounds.

The wait for treatment in the A&E can run into hours. Was Tom aware of that and did he feel that a fuss was being made over nothing and he'd be better off going home and sorting out the cut himself? He certainly didn't wish to go to hospital and told a police officer at the scene that he was happy to take responsibility for himself.

What happened next is still not known. An all-important few minutes that would change the Inglis family forever.

Tom didn't want to go to hospital but was persuaded to get into the ambulance. It set off.

The ambulance doors were opened at possibly as many as three times and Tom jumped or fell out. Later, Frances would struggle to believe that her son opened the doors and took the decision to jump out. She wondered what had transpired in the back of the ambulance, had Tom got involved in an argument, demanded that he be allowed out and been told no?

Whatever the truth behind his final few seconds in the ambulance as it travelled to the hospital, one thing is certain – Thomas did fall, and the momentum whipped his body around.

The vehicle was travelling at around thirty miles an hour, not a high speed but fast enough to cause catastrophic damage. Watching action films or TV shows, it is easy to imagine that jumping from a moving car isn't too difficult, that, by rolling to the side, the hero can dust himself off and walk away. But it is make-believe, a fantasy. A fall at speed cannot be controlled. Limbs might be broken, but of course a broken leg can heal. Far, far more seriously, leaving a moving vehicle can, and often does, cause someone to strike their head on the ground, on the hard tarmac or pavement.

The brain is highly vulnerable to impact injuries. Closed injuries are the most common; there may not be an open wound or fracture to the skull but if the head moves violently, billions of vital nerve fibres can be torn as the brain smashes from one side of the skull to the other. This is the worst case scenario.

An open or penetrating wound can look more alarming because of blood loss – head wounds bleed profusely as the head is well-serviced by the blood supply – but in fact the damage can be localised and relatively minor. Along with damage to nerve fibres, the real concern in fact comes with what is called the 'third injury', when a patient has been stabilised but the blood leaking from the bruised and delicate vessels in the brain starts causing it to swell.

The skull is designed to be a tough and unyielding space, but in trauma cases this rigidity is itself the danger. The build-up of internal pressure can restrict blood flow or cause terrible damage to soft brain tissue as it is forced against bone, and so it is crucial that this intracranial pressure is monitored carefully once a patient is admitted with head injuries.

Tom's head had struck the pavement, and severe head trauma was the first and foremost concern. He was rushed to Queen's Hospital in Romford and the police began the grim but essential task of informing his next of kin that he had been involved in an accident.

To open the door and find two police officers on the doorstep would alarm any parent, no matter the age of their child. The news was broken to Frances soon after seven in the morning. She was rushed to Queen's along with her youngest son, Michael, picking up Tom's other brother, Alex, on the way. Tom's father, also called Alex, arrived soon afterwards and together they gathered to sit at Tom's bedside in Intensive Care.

The shock to the family was considerable. Seeing Tom didn't in any way help them to grasp the reality of what had happened, but seemed only to add to their collective sense of confusion and disbelief. It seemed incredible that this damaged person wired up to machines and drips was their son and brother.

For Frances, the journey to the hospital had been one of deep anxiety but also of hope that her son's injuries could be quickly treated. Once in the hospital, however, she became gripped by profound distress. Something, she knew, was terribly wrong.

By the time she was joined by her ex-husband, her eldest son Alex sensed his mother was anguished in a way that he had never seen before. Doctors in charge of Tom's care told the family that he needed emergency surgery in order to lift a section of his skull and relieve the pressure on a bruised section of his brain. He would also need a tracheotomy, a tube inserted into his windpipe, to help him with his breathing.

Frances was distraught. She did not want her son to undergo the surgery. Her instincts screamed out to her that Tom was terribly ill and that surgery would only further mutilate him. She suspected that the surgeons wanted to operate so as to keep Tom alive at any cost lest it reflect badly on them and the emergency services. Looking at her son, she was no longer confident that he was 'alive' at all; it seemed to her that he had gone and only his broken body remained.

Tom's father and her son Alex tried to reason with Frances, and insisted that the operation should go ahead. The doctor present explained that without the surgery Tom could die, to which Frances replied, 'There are worse things than death.'

The shock and fear that families face when a loved one's life is in the balance can disorientate even the strongest of characters. Hospital staff endeavour to do all they can for seriously injured patients, but it isn't always possible that family members can be helped to cope with their sense of loss and panic. Added to the shock is a sense of helplessness, of being powerless because everything is out of their hands. They are reduced to acting as spectators watching the disintegrating life of a human being they knew so intimately.

Head trauma can induce coma and the Inglis family – as with any family in a similar situation – had to endure the many anxious hours that pass in waiting for Tom to show signs that he would regain consciousness. Perhaps then Frances's anguish would have some measure of relief . . .

After his operation, Frances sat with her unconscious son. He had staples in his head and was wired to machinery through a number of tubes. Tom's girlfriend, Danielle, arrived and she was overwhelmed by the sight of this figure and had to leave the room to be violently sick. Frances later said, 'I felt that Tom had died, I felt that I was looking at him and he had died.'

From the moment he was admitted to hospital, Tom had a constant stream of loved ones at his side: his father and brothers, his girlfriend, his aunts. But it was his mother who never missed a single day, and watched over him constantly. Yet the tiny flame of hope that was kindled when he finally began to stir was quickly dampened.

Tom's efforts to regain full and functioning consciousness were faltering. He began to open his eyes but was clearly disorientated. That in itself was hardly surprising, but Alex sensed that even when his brother made eye contact when he was spoken to, he still 'didn't seem fully conscious'. Like a newborn infant, he seemed unaware of the world around him except for passing moments and it was painful to watch him remain unable to engage with his loved ones. They were beyond his reach, beyond his broken mind.

If this was Tom, the real Tom, he would have tried to speak as soon as he had come round. He would have cracked a joke, tried to reassure his mum that he was okay. Even if struggling to speak, if this was Tom, his personality would have shone through. But he could not speak and, more significantly, he appeared unable to hold a thought.

On 10 July, a second decompression operation to remove more of his skull was carried out. The operations may have been life-saving necessities but an unfortunate result was severe disfigurement. Yet worse was to come. Tom started to fit.

Watching anyone suffering a fit is deeply distressing. The uncontrollably flailing limbs and convulsing body seem to mimic someone in the throes of extreme pain. At other times Tom would sweat profusely and appear panicked and unable to breathe. His mother, at his side, absorbed all his distress and began to torment herself with wondering why her son had been pulled back from the brink of death, only to be entombed in a body that seemed uncontrollable and violent and a mind that was beyond their reach.

Frances also watched as the tracheotomy tube that helped him breathe had to be cleared out using suction. She said, 'I could see the fear in Tom's eyes, the horror in Tom's eyes, every time they came to do it. How much more was he expected to endure?'

Raging between the grief of a thousand questions about why and how her bright and handsome son had been reduced to a shell was the nagging sense that she should help him, she should somehow relieve his pain and misery. She had to do something, she could not simply sit by and watch him unable to communicate and locked in agony, could she? For Frances, there was no respite. Waking or sleeping, her every thought was for Tom, and Alex grew concerned for her wellbeing; her anxiety over his brother seemed to have unbalanced her.

When the family questioned the medical team that was caring for Tom they were told that the prognosis was not unpromising. He could begin to show improvements in brain function over the longer term. Try as she might, Frances found it a struggle to believe that her son would recover.

In the days after Tom had been admitted to Queen's, Frances spoke to one of her neighbours, Sharon Robinson. By that time, everyone knew of the accident and were full of sympathy for Frances and the Inglis family. It was a horrible twist of fate that a young man in his prime should now be fighting for his life.

Sharon saw Frances and her heart went out to her. What can a neighbour say at such a terrible time? But the conversation took a turn Sharon never expected. Frances asked if her friend knew where she could buy some heroin. Pure heroin. Not quite able to believe what she'd been asked, Sharon asked what Frances meant. It was simple, Frances told her. She wanted 'to put it in her son to end his misery'.

Sharon was upset to see her friend in such distress but knew it would be sensible to call the police. If something did happen and she had not alerted those who could help Frances and protect Tom, it would be unforgivable. The police duly arrived and spoke to Frances, who broke down. They took her home and spent time with her, attempting to calm and reassure her.

The strain of the last ten days had been considerable, and she admitted that she had asked her neighbour about purchasing an illegal drug but stressed that she had done so only in a fit of anger. Sensing that this was a mother lost in grief, the police referred Frances to a counsellor.

Adjusting to loss is overwhelming and often frightening. All moorings are lost as the bereaved one pitches from one fraught emotion to another – from numbness to fury, from fear to remorse, and even to guilt. Perhaps she should have stopped Tom going out, Frances thought; should have known that something was going to happen. Totally irrational thoughts that rise to the surface when tragedy and grief overtake reason.

Had Tom died on that first night, there would at least have been a structure to Frances's sense of loss, something 'normal' that everyone in her life could understand even if they could not measure the depth of her grief. But this was different. Tom was 'alive' and no one seemed to understand Frances at all.

Summer had come and gone. It was early September and the schools were preparing to re-open.

September feels like the start of a new year, a rhythm that never leaves no matter the age of the child. Sports kits and uniforms were washed and ironed, children were measured for new shoes, lunch boxes and stationery were assembled; all the hectic but humdrum tasks that come with motherhood. But not all mothers.

Frances, too, should have been preparing to return to her college nursing course, but she was alone and adrift. Her only focus in life was Tom and her vigil at his side.

It was approaching two months since his accident and she was more convinced than ever that he was being kept alive artificially. Her greatest concern was that being unable to communicate, her son was trapped in pain and suffering and no one was helping him because no one could hear him.

Alex was increasingly concerned for his mother. He hoped that Tom might start to improve, but whenever the subject was raised Frances told Alex that not only did she not believe that Tom could get any better, but that it was cruel to keep him alive and in pain.

Frances had lost faith in the medical interventions her son was subjected to. Her constant presence at Tom's side was exhausting, and Alex suspected that it was preventing his mother from thinking calmly or rationally. Her worry that Tom might be in pain was becoming an obsession.

It is very difficult to predict the ultimate outcome of serious head injuries for a patient. The doctors caring for Tom remained hopeful; they noted gradual improvements in his responses. Tom's surgeon Mr Ragu Vindlacheruvu, knew that while it was possible for Tom eventually to recover sufficiently to live independently, it was equally possible that he wouldn't – that he could die as an in-patient.

So wide is the variance and scope for deterioration or recovery that doctors have to be honest about how little is certain. They did not wish the family to give up hope, but it was clearly evident that there would be no overnight miracles.

When Ragu Vindlacheruvu visited Tom's bedside on 4 September, he was happy with his patient's overall health. No matter how experienced they are, medical staff never become inured to what they see and what they have to deal with. On a good day, a child might sit up and smile for the first time after head injuries caused in a car crash; on another day, a patient who has shown signs of recovery can be lost forever. As a consultant in the high dependency unit, Mr Vindlacheruvu had seen the best and the worst of outcomes but was quietly hopeful that, given time, Tom would rally.

Walking into Tom's room that September day, he later remembered, his patient looked fine. He said hello to Frances and realised that she had ignored his greeting. He decided not to dwell on it, Frances was attending to Tom and he didn't wish to interfere.

It was later that same day that a nurse sounded the alarm. Tom was not breathing and had a strange pallor. As the crash team rushed to the room, she began frantic efforts to re-start his heart. But Thomas Inglis was dead, his heart at a standstill, his damaged brain starved of oxygen. As the seconds and minutes ticked by, the attitude of the crash team remained one of fixed determination – if their patient's heart would start pumping once more, there would still be hope.

And it happened. After a frantic few minutes, Tom's heart suddenly thudded back to life and began to beat once more.

The Inglis family would have to be told about Tom's setback, of course, but with the crisis dealt with one of the team remembered that two days earlier Tom's father had asked staff to watch Frances if she were on her own with Tom. It was an odd request. After the critical incident, Mr Inglis talked about it with Alex. Officially, Tom had suffered a heart attack, but with heavy hearts, both men wondered if Frances had tried to take matters into her own hands.

Alex Inglis Sr asked the hospital to run tests on his son's blood. He thought it might be possible that Tom had been poisoned. The subsequent toxicology report revealed high levels of heroin in Tom's system, probably administered via the tracheotomy that was helping him breathe.

The police were called. Alex admitted that he and his father suspected that Frances was going to 'try and do something', adding 'She just seemed to talk about it a lot more, trying to get people to agree that Thomas wasn't getting better.'

The nurse in charge of the ward at Queen's, Sister Maria Curtain, told police that Mr Inglis asked her, 'Do you think that she [Frances] had anything to do with this?' He had confided to the Sister that Frances had been researching euthanasia on the internet – a fact he only discovered when she asked one of her sons to clear the cache on her search engine.

When Frances was told that her son had survived, she said simply, 'Oh God.'

Frances was arrested on suspicion of attempted murder and detectives searched her home. There, they found notes stored under the stairs, one of which read:

People keep saying Tom isn't suffering. How do they know? Can they know the terror of knowing you cannot control anything anymore? Can they know the agony of being denied pain relief just to see his reaction? Without my begging and pleading Tom would just have been left to suffer. How can I trust such people?

49

She denied trying to kill Tom. Interviewed by detectives she said, 'I want my son to live. I want my son to get better. I want my son to recover.'

It was not felt that Frances represented a threat to anyone else and she was allowed out on bail. However, her release came with the strict condition that she was not to be in contact with Thomas, and a photograph of her was placed behind the nursing station on the ward at Queen's. She was not to approach her son.

Now Frances would have to wait, alone and distraught, for her trial date. And while she waited, her only and every thought was for her son and what might be happening to him.

In another of the typed notes found by the detectives, Frances had written, *What if he is in a dark and terrifying place?* If he was, he would continue to be so without his mother at his side.

3

At What Cost?

—

The quiet hours pass. Often they are slow and sometimes they are mercifully uneventful but they pass; even when they are filled with watchful anxiety, they pass. Time moves on.

Caring for a chronically ill child has a disorientating effect on time. When sickness worsens, the minutes are measured out fitfully as mothers wait anxiously for signs of improvement and for analgesics to begin to relieve pain. Each hour is fought for.

When the illness is in abeyance, a day can drag and yet parents can note with dismay that in fact the months have accumulated unnoticed and years have passed. Friends' lives have moved on, other children they once knew are now adults and planning families of their own. The normal rhythms of life have slipped away.

The Gilderdales' devotion to Lynn never wavered. Kay and Richard were determined to do all they could to support their daughter, to help her overcome the myriad ailments that further weakened her slight frame, and to focus on the future. But for how long? It was a question

Kay did not want to ask herself. Her commitment to Lynn was absolute and unwavering, she would remain at her side forever and a day if necessary, though she believed Lynn would get well again.

For carers, a stasis eventually sets in, a terrible inertia, within which they manage the day-to-day requirements of feeding, cleaning, medicating, and providing companionship, but the memory of how life once was in normal times imperceptibly fades away.

Lynn was not getting better. Every system of her body was affected and she required twenty-four-hour care. Kay was encouraged to take time off for herself but found it impossible because thoughts of her daughter's suffering would impede her efforts to switch off. The longest she ever allowed herself to stay away, even when visiting relatives in Ireland, was two days. And besides, she missed her daughter too much. She greatly valued their time together and still counted her blessings that Lynn was a fighter; a funny girl who could still make the family laugh out loud with her views on the world.

It is easy to imagine that Lynn's life had become little more than the four walls that surrounded her, and in many ways it had. She was bedbound and in constant pain, and although medication helped, she suffered persistent stomach pain and headaches. But through the form of sign language she had developed, she did communicate with her family and Kay felt honoured to care for her.

Remarkably, for one who had lost all semblance of a healthy life so young, Lynn never complained. Kay would later say, 'She didn't complain, she might lie and cry in pain sometimes but she didn't complain.' But Lynn did continue worrying about the effect her illness was having on her mother's life. Richard and brother Steve also helped to look after her but the main burden fell squarely on Kay's shoulders. An intercom in Lynn's room was always switched on so that Lynn could tap it, which allowed Kay to listen out for her when going about necessary household tasks such as the laundry, or preparing the numerous array of medications required to sustain Lynn. Twice a week a carer would come so that Kay could do the shopping and any other outside chores. Those were the only times she left the house.

Improvements were made to Lynn's room. Her other 'companions' came to be, at one stage, two cats, whom she adored. As time went on, she was also able to listen to music and use a small, hand-held computer.

On her better days, she would look at magazines with her mother and they'd order clothes through catalogues. Clothes that she planned to wear once she was better and could walk from the room. Beautiful dresses that spoke of a world that existed just beyond her view and yet so tantalisingly close. Lynn imagined parties and the anticipation all young women feel when they plan what they'd like to wear. She dreamed of being invited out to dinner and walking under the street lights of a busy city arm-in-arm with a boyfriend.

It was deeply painful to acknowledge that life was just beyond her grasp. So much had been lost, and now the tally was no longer in months but in years. Lynn's father, Richard, recalled how 'we used to sit on the beach and look at Lynn and her brother enjoying themselves and we would think how lucky we were to have such fit and healthy children . . . It's where she was free and before she knew what pain was, and hospital; and sickness.' Now all that was left seemed to be the drift of interminable illness and gradual decline.

Kay was desperate to believe that it didn't always have to be this way. Slowly, she had come to learn more and more about ME and its impact on sufferers and their families. She knew that people *did* get better, *did* improve and manage their illness, with only the occasional setback and period of extended bed rest. Many returned to work, picked up the pieces of a life that had left them behind, and began a new chapter.

All of this was encouraging, and ME support networks began to emerge. The internet of course was a massive boost. It allowed people, no matter how isolated, to reach out and find support and advice. Isolation was a very real and very difficult issue to manage. Ignorance surrounding the condition was still widespread, and it was not only sufferers but also their carers who were out of sight and without voice.

When people did emerge from a bout of severe ME, they very often met with the uncharitable opinion that their condition had been brought on because of a character flaw, a psychological fault that could be treated if they were disciplined enough. Such misconceptions were probably fed by the fact that most people only meet those with ME once they are already in recovery, at their best, and back in society. Shoulders were shrugged and eyebrows raised about 'chronic fatigue'.

Such ill-informed remarks can give offence or cause hurt. Kay told of one occasion when someone from social services came to meet Lynn and 'said she did not believe in ME, but it was obvious how ill she was'. As if the condition wasn't real and yet Lynn was happy to lie in bed, her veins collapsing through constant administration of drugs and her years slipping away from her. What's more, the steroids Lynn had to take to combat adrenal failure caused her bones to thin.

In truth, a quarter of all ME sufferers are so badly affected that they become housebound, bedbound, or unable to move without a wheelchair. Lynn's illness was pernicious and particularly virulent. Kay began to campaign for others with the condition and to speak out. She never saw herself in the role of campaigner but if Lynn could be so strong and brave, she was sure that she could overcome her natural reserve to try and help alter perceptions of the illness.

❋

Despite Lynn's best efforts to be positive and imagine a time when she would be well, more setbacks were on the way. In her late teens, she began to suffer ovarian failure after her body stopped producing oestrogen. Although she went onto HRT subsequently, she contracted severe osteoporosis linked to the lack of hormones.

It was a devastating further disability. Even as a child, Lynn had always spoken with confidence about one day being a mother and now that possibility was taken from her. She had already lost so much. Her teenage years, her education, all the experiences and privileges of being young and carefree. For the family, too, it was hard to embrace what lay ahead, but Kay was determined that life had to go on and that even now, her daughter's situation was not without hope.

For Lynn's eighteenth birthday Kay made eighteen little presents, which she wrapped individually and placed inside a biscuit tin. Then she iced the tin and placed eighteen candles on it, as if on a cake. When she showed it to her daughter Lynn smiled, pleased, but said she could not eat it. Then Kay showed her what the cake really was.

These were some of the small moments and memories mother and daughter cherished. It was by now too poignant to recall Lynn as she had once been, and too painful to think of a future that was being denied to her. It was safest perhaps to focus on what lay ahead of them each day and to hope and pray that, slowly, the illness would abate.

The millennium came and went. Kay thought how Lynn's friends, now young women in their early twenties, would have celebrated; she wondered whether they were enjoying careers, or were thinking about setting up a home with a boyfriend, or even planning their weddings . . .

Sadly, her own marriage was unravelling. While she and Richard remained on the best of terms, a distance had grown up between them which they couldn't seem to bridge. Kay didn't feel that this was connected to Lynn's illness, and after they divorced in 2002 Lynn remained at the centre of both their worlds. Richard still called his daughter his best friend, and he and Kay took a shared delight in the way Lynn engaged with the world on her own terms.

Kay said, 'You would think that somebody who has been removed from society would be very backward in a lot of things because she has not had much input for such a long time, but now Lynn is right on the ball about everything.' And Kay was right. Her daughter was bright, very intelligent, and who knows what she could have achieved if ME had not so cruelly attacked her.

When she was feeling at her best Lynn could use the internet, and she eventually began a blog using a false name. It was through the blog that the depth of her character shone through. On some levels this was harder to bear, knowing how happily she would embrace the world if she were given the chance. On her better days, she would joke about liking Robbie Williams and manage to look at clothes online. She would say that she hadn't come this far, through so many years of suffering, to give up now. And Kay believed her, believed in her determination and grit. Asked what she would do should she recover her health, Lynn would carefully fold her arms together and make a slight rocking motion, as if holding a baby.

But on the worst days, the long accumulation of restless nights and weeks of setbacks, it was as if Lynn were entombed. 'If someone dies,' said Kay, 'you mourn them, then you get to a stage where you know that person is gone and you move on.

'But she is neither one nor the other. She is stuck in that room, not dead, but not alive properly. It is an awful place to be. If I didn't believe, and she didn't believe, that one day she would get better then I don't think it would be right for her to go on suffering like this for a whole lifespan of seventy or eighty years.'

Time stretched endlessly before them and the chances of recovery receded.

In October 2005 Lynn was admitted to the Conquest Hospital in Hastings to have her Hickman line, an intravenous catheter, changed under local anaesthetic.

During the procedure, her lung was punctured and an

artery was damaged, resulting in one lung filling with blood and the other filling halfway. She was placed on life support and transferred to King's College Hospital in London. There she remained unconscious for three weeks and her family feared that she would not survive. Her last words to her parents had been, 'Goodbye, I love you.'

But Lynn woke up. There was relief all round, but something in Lynn had changed. She was adamant that she did not wish to be resuscitated if she were ever to fall so ill again. She now felt that she was a prisoner of her condition; a prisoner with a positive attitude, perhaps, but one who possibly had just had enough.

After regaining consciousness, Lynn had remained in hospital for three months, part of the time in intensive care, part in high dependency. When she came home, the Gilderdales' family doctor visited. She noted that Lynn felt that her 'body was broken'. The doctor did not doubt that the illness had left Lynn with unimaginable physical difficulties.

It cannot be surprising that anyone, having suffered in such a condition for fourteen years, would question why they were still hanging on to a semblance of a life and question why medical intervention strove for life at any cost. But doctors swear an oath to preserve life; judgements as to 'quality of life' are subjective and not for doctors to make. So who does make the judgement and what control do we have over our deaths?

Until that point, Lynn had talked about her family as a team. Now, as her parents continued to fight every minute of every day to improve her condition, she began to question what was possible.

The fear she had once felt about hospitals returned and she resolved that, should she be reduced to her recent hospitalised condition again, it would end differently. Richard, who understood his daughter when she came to describe her body as broken, said, 'It was the turning point. She said that she never ever wanted to be put on a life support machine ever again. She became more determined that she didn't want to go into hospital ever again. She then started generally introducing us to the fact that she decided she never wanted to be resuscitated again.'

A Do Not Resuscitate note was placed on Lynn's medical notes at her own wish. She later went a step further and directed that a living will should be drafted, in which she stated her wish not to be resuscitated or subjected to any medical intervention if her quality of life remained so poor. The will, drawn up by a solicitor, included the following words from Lynn: 'I wish it to be understood I fear degeneration and indignity far more than I fear death.'

For Richard, it was very difficult to listen to his daughter resign herself to such a fate. Hardest of all was when she would look at him with a knowing expression in her eyes and say, 'Look, it's never going to go away, Dad.' He realised that his beautiful daughter was moving beyond the 'team', that she was dealing with a newer, harder set of feelings and beliefs. She had made up her own mind that she couldn't carry on.

He knew Lynn would not have arrived at such a position lightly; she would have thought about things very deeply and examined every eventuality. Her battle now was not only the illness itself, with all that that implied, but to make her parents understand that if she were to deteriorate further (she also had heart, kidney, liver and thyroid problems by this stage), she didn't want medical intervention at all – she would choose to die.

Richard had to start seeing the situation through his daughter's eyes. What was her life like? She couldn't eat, she couldn't drink. She had been admitted to hospital fifty or sixty times. Not only were her hopes for the future cruelly taken – she couldn't have children and her brittle bones made it unlikely that she could walk – but she also lived in constant pain and the fear that a new bout of illness could leave her with brain damage and placed into long-term care.

'Home was all she had,' Richard would later say. 'It was the only place where she felt safe and secure. She knew that everybody in the home environment would fight every minute of every day for her.'

He spoke of his daughter's gratitude for her parents' support: 'She said on many occasions that if it hadn't been for her mum and her family she would have died years ago.'

After her last setback, however, maybe home was no longer enough. Kay always fought to stay positive for their daughter. Inwardly, Richard thought but did not want to admit that Lynn would never get better. As time passed, she spoke openly to her parents about her body, asking them to accept that it had 'broken down'. This was not a sign of depression but of Lynn's resolve, of her determination that her parents accept that optimism was no longer enough. Richard asked her why she hated her life, and she replied that she could see no end to her suffering. His usual assertions, his remarks of 'just hang on in there' no longer lit up his daughter's eyes.

In 2007, Richard became aware that his daughter had contacted Dignitas, the Swiss-based euthanasia group. Lynn spoke to him about it, but Richard was opposed to the idea of her using their services, saying, 'I didn't want the thought of my daughter going somewhere like that.' They talked about it regularly even though, in reality, it would have been impossible to take Lynn that distance without her suffering further; even lifting her risked breaking a bone. It was also, Lynn felt, a cold and heartless way to manage her death – she wanted to remain at home where she felt cherished, and where she felt safe.

One of the few items which afforded Lynn any degree of privacy was her handheld computer which she used to contact other people with ME and illnesses such as cancer and multiple sclerosis. She also used her handheld computer to access the *LiveJournal* forum, on which she detailed her desire to end her life. In one extract, she described her '. . . miserable excuse for life. I'm tired, so very, very tired. I can't keep hanging on to an ever-diminishing hope that I might one day be well again.' In another section, she told how she was 'tired and my spirit is broken' and how she would grab an opportunity to leave the world 'with both hands'.

Slowly but inevitably, Kay and Richard had to accept that Lynn was adamant. It was not right of them to want to keep her with them for their sakes alone; their daughter had the right to say that she no longer wanted to suffer. Richard eventually said to her, 'I understand why you don't want to be here. I don't want you to go but I understand.' It was a heartbreaking admission.

Fathers will give anything of themselves to protect their children. Admitting that events are beyond their control and that their wishes may stand in direct opposition to those of their child is emotionally punishing.

It was in 2007 that Lynn made a suicide attempt, injecting herself with morphine. Her attempt had failed, but Richard guessed what had happened when he walked into her bedroom to find her looking very sleepy.

The Gilderdales were now left to face the dreadful truth – their daughter could neither live nor die; she was trapped, and she no longer wished to carry on. All attempts to recover some sort of balance, to find some sort of focus outside the illness foundered. Lynn had had little or no control over her life for many, many years. She had fought hard, she had endured more than anyone could have expected of her. Now her mind was made up. She had found a new and different type of courage – the courage to say 'enough'.

Christmas was approaching, a time for families and the giving of gifts. Richard asked Lynn what she would like: 'She just shrugged her shoulders and looked away from me. I knew what she was saying.'

4

The Last Goodbye

All children are different. Even two of the same gender, brought up in the same household, can turn out to be extraordinarily diverse characters. Perhaps we are all born with a certain template, a fixed and stubborn core of self that does not alter no matter what we experience or undergo.

When Frances Inglis thought of her son Thomas, she remembered what kind of boy he had always been. From the very outset, he was hardy and independent, fearless even. He loved and looked up to his brother Alex, but he certainly didn't entertain for a minute the idea that he would stand in Alex's shadow. Or anybody else's. Tom was his own man from the very start and he hated anyone making a fuss of him.

An all-boy household can be a loud and boisterous environment; boys are typically quick to anger, but also quick to move on and forgive. They see the world as something to capture and explore and Tom was no different. When he developed a passion for something, nothing would stop him from throwing himself into it wholeheartedly.

Frances recalled how when Tom was twelve he hit upon a new hobby – fishing. She didn't have the first idea about the world of fishing but, as always, Tom was undeterred. He read and researched what equipment he would need, made decisions about what he'd like to buy, got hold of the various bits and pieces, and set off for the river.

He spent a winter by himself at the side of the river and was never put off by his failure to catch a single fish. It was his passion, and all he needed was to be thinking and doing things for himself. That was when he was at his happiest.

After he left school, a career as a pipe-fitter suited his personality too. Although part of a team, his role allowed him to work independently, making assessments and decisions about how best to solve an engineering or logistical problem in piping systems. It is not to be confused with plumbing; pipe-fitters work on industrial and large-scale heating or cooling systems that require a high degree of precision as different alloys are fused together.

Frances was proud of her boys. Alex enjoyed his work as a chef and Tom loved his job. Everything seemed to be going so well for him; he had met Danielle and was very happy. It was all a mother could hope for, for her son, a man of twenty-one.

The fallout from the failed attempt to end Tom's life was devastating. The family were in shock, and no one could come to terms with Tom's accident or the impact it had had on Frances.

For her friends and neighbours, events were difficult to believe. Frances had spent years helping the sick, the disabled and disadvantaged. Her friend Pauline Greenwood, who met her through a church-based amateur dramatics group, said she would watch her friend 'in pieces' outside her son's hospital, and eventually took Frances to see a GP to get help. 'I worried about her mental health,' she said. 'She was a shell. She aged a lot.'

This Frances was unrecognisable as the woman Pauline knew, the woman who loved ballroom dancing and whose only vice was cigarettes. The woman who had begun a series of training courses to help others and who, by 2000, was working as a community support worker in Barking and Dagenham. That was the Frances whose co-worker Gillian Morris described as 'a special person and a good mum,' while another friend, Lorna Baker, observed that she 'did not have a nasty bone in her body'.

Frances had gone on to become a learning support assistant for pupils with profound learning difficulties at Newbridge School, Ilford. The deputy-head, Mary Dunne, said, 'Frankie left us to train as a mental health professional and if I could have her back I would.'

Undoubtedly, she was well-loved and much respected, but now no one seemed able to reach her. Her every thought was for Tom, whose life she believed was over because he was trapped in a body that did not work and which caused him pain. Had her experience of working with those with disabilities also framed her thoughts about what Tom would have found intolerable? Did she feel that she would be failing her son if she didn't help him, thereby creating an impossible burden for both of them? But what could she now do . . .?

Tom was being transferred. He had been moved once already, to Northwick Park in Middlesex, but this move was to take him to the privately run Gardens Neuro Centre, a fifty-two-bed neurological services centre on the Rivers Hospital site at Sawbridgeworth in East Hertfordshire. The Centre provided twenty-four-hour nursing care, and therapy services for adults with complex neurological conditions.

According to the Centre's website, together with the sixty-bed Jacobs Neuro Unit on the same site, the facility existed to 'assist recovery wherever possible and specialise in slow-stream rehabilitation. Emphasis is placed on maximising each individual's abilities, comfort and quality of life.'

'Quality of life' is the term that jars with many families who must pick up the pieces after a catastrophic accident or illness. Who defines what is or is not 'quality' when the patients can't speak for themselves?

The transfer went ahead in May 2008. The staff were

informed that Frances Inglis was barred from visiting her son, but no photograph of her was issued to the nurses in order to enforce this.

It was not until six months later that Frances had everything in place. It was November, the evenings were dark and cold, and she believed that it was time to help her son once and for all. She had always been there for him, always been there for her boys, and her nerve must not fail her now.

Her trial for the attempt on Tom's life was pending. She had limited time, and now a new situation was developing which convinced her that she must prepare in earnest. That situation was that Alex and his father had begun to discuss the possibility of applying for a court order to allow the withdrawal of nutrition and hydration from Tom – a means of bringing about his death which was entirely legal.

To Frances, this was a horrific solution. Such a decision might be within the law but, effectively, it meant watching her son die of starvation and thirst. She could imagine him crying from thirst but being unable to move or be heard as he slowly wasted away. It was too much. In truth, it was barbaric.

And so she decided to lay her plans. Everything would have to be carefully thought through to the last detail, every eventuality assessed. She could not risk failing her son again.

Before Tom's accident, Frances had had no idea where to

obtain heroin. It was ludicrous. Once, she would not have even known where to start looking. Asking her neighbour that first time had been a mistake, and she now took to waiting outside the train station, hoping that it would become obvious who was likely to know how to buy the drug. It was a ludicrous and risky way of doing things, but she eventually got what she needed. Ten small wraps of heroin.

Next, she thought about planning for her home and family in the event of her absence. At no stage did Frances imagine that she would escape from the police. She was ready to account fully for her actions, knowing that what she was about to do, she did with the best intentions, no matter what the courts might think.

She carefully compiled instructions for her family, including how to pay the bills, and reminders to feed Max, the family dog, with chicken wings from Asda; she asked that they ensure that he had a supply of freshly changed water in his bowl.

She had not seen Tom for about a year, an absence that she had found intolerably painful. Now she spoke to her ex-husband and he agreed that she could visit Tom with him. They travelled together to the Centre three or four times before the visit that would end her son's life.

On that last critical day, 21 November, Frances drove north to the hospital in her ex-husband's Ford Mondeo. She had learnt the codes to get in the door at Sawbridgeworth and when she arrived there she posed as an aunt of Tom's, giving her name as Atkins.

She was quite composed: she knew that this was her last and only chance. And she had made a promise to herself and a promise to Tom that she would release him from the prison of his ruined body and shattered mind. She went to his room and left the door open because she had noted that the doors to the patients' rooms were never shut.

Sitting with her son for the last time, perhaps thinking back over the life they had known in happier times and how proud she was of the man he had become, Frances told Tom that she loved him. Then she opened her handbag and took out the syringe and the heroin. Steadying her nerve and the turmoil in her mind, she injected Tom in the thigh and arms. Tom, who was fed by a tube into his stomach and was unable to speak, slowly began to process the 'ten little parcels' of heroin. She held him and told him that everything would be fine.

She was alone with Tom for almost half an hour before anyone came. When a nurse did arrive to give Tom his medication Frances screamed, 'Not now, I've got HIV and if you come in here I'll start spitting at you.' She was so afraid that he would be resuscitated once more that she had to have enough time with him; this time she *had* to be sure. She put a chair and the oxygen tank in front of the door in an attempt to block it and, using superglue, tried to disable the lock.

Tom seemed very peaceful. This was the death she had wished for him, a serene end. No more hoists, no more tubes, no more indignities and no more pain.

The staff outside the door were frantic while Frances sat with her son for the last time. What would happen to her next did not trouble her. Her only thought was to release Tom. She held his hand; a hand that she had first kissed twenty-two years ago. And then it was time to say goodbye to her bold and beautiful son.

5

'Please can you come now.
Be careful. Don't rush.'

———

There are certain phrases used by police which, over a period of time, become familiar to the public, part of everyday English whose meaning is instantly understood.

One such phrase was spoken by Chief Inspector Heather Keating of the Sussex Police Force when she said, on 8 December 2008, 'This is a very tragic incident, but we are not looking for anyone else in connection with it.'

The 'incident' she was referring to was the death of Lynn Gilderdale, and the obvious inference to be drawn was that police had 'got their man' – or, in this case, their woman. In case there should be any doubt, a spokesman for Sussex police stated that 'A 54-year-old woman from Stonegate, arrested on suspicion of murder, has been interviewed and bailed to return on March 6th.'

Police had been called to Lynn's home at eight-thirty a.m. on Thursday, 4 December, and her mother Kay had been bailed the following day.

One newspaper spelt out clearly what they thought had happened:

A mother who nursed her daughter for 17 years with the disease ME has been arrested on suspicion of her murder following what is believed to have been a 'mercy killing'.

Police sources revealed that Lynn Gilderdale, 31, died from a massive overdose of morphine after attempting suicide with the same drug at least twice during her battle with the debilitating condition. Detectives arrested her mother Kay, 54, over suspicions that she helped administer the fatal dose after watching her daughter suffer since she was fourteen

The story started to feed through news channels, but it wasn't just the police who were issuing pronouncements; Lynn's family made a statement too, but of a rather more moving nature:

Lynn was young, beautiful, loving and caring. At the age of fourteen years she was struck down by ME – an illness greatly misunderstood – and as a result, suffered the stigma attached to this dreadful illness. She fought long and hard for seventeen years with immense bravery, enduring constant pain and sickness.

They described briefly her health history and how she fell ill, deteriorated, and lost the power of speech.

Prior to her illness, which left her paralysed, unable to speak, eat or drink and, until recently, no memory, she was an active healthy teenager full of life's dreams. She enjoyed sailing, swimming, cycling and was an accomplished musician.

Her family praised and admired Lynn for her courage, which she showed to the end.

She was a much-loved daughter, sister and granddaughter who, despite her illness, always gave love and support to others.

Lynn's family said her death would leave a massive void in their lives – and the love she gave so unreservedly would be missed every minute of the day.

Despite the huge and terrible loss, the family vowed to continue campaigning for better understanding of ME. Even then, it seemed, some were questioning how 'chronic fatigue'could be so extreme and debilitating.

Against a backdrop of ignorance and misunderstanding about the illness itself, the Gilderdales also had to contend with a rising tide in public and press opinion about 'mercy killings', even though Kay had never believed that the description was one that fitted her actions. In fact, almost immediately following the news of Lynn's death, even though the exact circumstances were not revealed until many months later in court, there was no shortage of opinion on the events in the Gilderdale home.

A private tragedy had become a national talking point for commentators, and those looking for law reform as well as those opposed to any form of the right to die, were weighing in on all sides. For Kay, the loss of her daughter was something she struggled with every day. It was not her own fate that troubled her, but her aching sense of loss now that Lynn had gone and the painful void that had been left by her passing.

While Kay waited to hear if she would be tried for murder, the debate about whether it can ever be right to help someone take their own life raged on. A reform to existing laws could, it was argued, at least provide sufferers and their families with a choice about how to end their lives. But, ran the counter argument, the same law could also be misused by families or individuals looking to 'rid' themselves of a troublesome burden.

How a law can be drafted to fully protect the needs of the vulnerable is far from clear cut, but campaigners are quick – and correct – to point out that the status quo has not entirely prevented the occurrence of assisted deaths.

Professor Clive Seale of Brunel University estimates that about nine hundred deaths per year in the UK are assisted by doctors. As the law is clear, a greater understanding of what doctors are or are not doing in 'end of life' management is important. In 2006 Professor Seale conducted the first survey among doctors about euthanasia. In total, 857 medical practitioners responded to the survey, which guaranteed anonymity so that responses were more likely to be given freely and honestly.

What the survey revealed was startling. The overwhelming majority of doctors, some eighty-two per cent, did not wish to see the law changed so as to allow medical involvement in euthanasia or assisted suicide. Yet these same doctors had played a part in 'end of life decisions'. Thirty per cent had sanctioned 'non-treatment' decisions, for example the withholding or withdrawing of treatment. And a further thirty-two per cent had prescribed the 'alleviation of symptoms with possibly life-shortening effect'.

For those who have been involved with the protracted complications brought on by a terminal illness in a friend or relative, this high-level use of pain-relieving drugs will be familiar and the risk that the drug will hasten the end of life is an ever-present factor.

Doctors are aware of the need to help people end their lives with a degree of control and dignity, yet it is important to note that not a single incident of 'physician-assisted suicide' was recorded in the survey results.

In summarising his findings, Professor Seale underlined the distinctions that doctors make about patient care:

'We have a very strong ethos of providing excellent palliative care in the UK, reflected in the finding that doctors in the UK are willing to make other kinds of decisions that prioritise the comfort of patients, without striving to preserve life at the cost of suffering.

'The results suggest that providing the best kind of patient care is a major driver behind medical decision making.'

Yet the decisions that doctors make do not always sit easily with the families who are left to deal with the wishes of their loved ones, whose lives have become defined by pain and suffering, as Lynn Gilderdale's had done.

There was much sympathy for the Gilderdales. Jane Colby, executive director of the Young ME Sufferers Trust and author of a number of books raising awareness of the severity of ME, had in the past spoken at length with Kay Gilderdale about the problems Lynn had encountered after she was taken into hospital. In Ms Colby's 1996 book, *ME: The New Plague*, Lynn's treatment was described, albeit anonymously.

Ms Colby, who fell ill with ME herself in 1985, and was still hampered by its effects, had worked with doctors in Britain and the United States to try and prove that those effects are caused by a virus she believes is similar to polio.

'You would not know how bad it was until you have seen somebody in that situation and had cared for somebody with it,' she said. 'You feel as if you have been poisoned, you are in pain constantly, you stink because of the sweat coming off you.

'It is dreadful. We are all devastated and our thoughts are with the [Gilderdale] family at this time.'

As well as working with Ms Colby to raise awareness of ME, Kay and Lynn were heavily involved with the 25% ME

Group, which was set up to provide support for the most severely afflicted sufferers. They were also, for a time, members of the Kent and Sussex ME Society whose chairman, Colin Barton, fundraised with Lynn's father, Richard, on several occasions.

'In Lynn we have a very brave young lady,' Barton said. 'She worked tirelessly for years, making the public aware of how severe the illness can be. The family have always done all they possibly can to help the cause of ME. The mother was a very caring woman who did all she could for Lynn.'

Both national and local newspapers carried letters from those who had suffered from ME, or from those who cared for sufferers, all of them pointing out the pain the Gilderdale family must have endured. One to *The Times* said: 'My sister died of this disease on November 25 2005. A post-mortem revealed the extent of her real physical illness. She suffered unnecessarily because a physical illness was treated as a mental one. How many more deaths will it take to change the way ME is treated?'

The police appeared to remain detached from the heartfelt outpourings of sympathy and the messages sent to the Gilderdales, and to the wider debate that was being conducted in the press. From their standpoint, they had a job to do, and how they did it was dictated by the law and investigative procedures.

In early March 2009, Sussex Police said it had extended Kay's bail until Tuesday, 7 April, for further investigation to be conducted. Only nine days later, on 16 April, came the sensational news that Kay Gilderdale was to be charged with attempted murder.

The decision had been made and it came down to Derek Frame, a Crown Prosecution Service lawyer, to explain: 'I have advised Sussex Police that there is sufficient evidence and it is in the public interest to charge Kathleen Gilderdale with the attempted murder of her daughter Lynette.

'In reviewing the evidence in this case, I also considered the offences of murder and assisted suicide. In order to support a charge of murder, the prosecution would have to prove that Mrs Gilderdale's actions significantly contributed to her daughter's death.

'There was insufficient evidence to prove this. In relation to assisted suicide, whilst this offence was considered, I decided that a charge of attempted murder more accurately reflected Mrs Gilderdale's actions and intentions.'

Kay was given conditional bail, and Brighton magistrates ordered her to appear at Lewes Crown Court on 30 April 2009. The police issued a brief statement:

'Kathleen Gilderdale, 54, of Stonegate, has been charged that between December 2 and December 4 2008, she attempted to murder Lynn Gilderdale, who was found dead at her home in Stonegate, near Heathfield, on December 4 last year.'

The Gilderdale family were appalled. Shortly afterwards, they issued their own statement:

'Following the decision yesterday by the Crown Prosecution Service to charge Kay Gilderdale with the attempted murder of her daughter Lynn, her entire family wish to express their extreme disappointment and sadness regarding this course of action and reiterate their continuing and unconditional support for Kay during these difficult times.

'Her family and friends will continue to work towards ensuring that Kay is recognised as the dedicated and loving mother of Lynn, who cared unreservedly for her daughter over so many years. Their hope is that this recognition will result in a quick and compassionate conclusion in the coming weeks.'

At Lewes Crown Court on that final day of April, it was alleged that Kay attempted to murder Lynn over the course of some thirty hours in early December 2008. Bespectacled, and wearing a grey suit and purple top, Kay did not enter a plea during the brief preliminary hearing. She was granted conditional bail to appear at the same court for a plea and case management hearing on 3 July.

Slowly the weeks passed as Kay and her family waited anxiously for the case to grind on to its next hearing. On 3 July, during a brief court appearance, Kay Gilderdale spoke only to confirm her name and enter her plea. She admitted the charge of aiding and abetting the suicide of her daughter, but denied the charge of attempted murder.

But her not guilty pleas were rejected by the Crown Prosecution Service, even though Judge Richard Brown invited the CPS to drop the other two charges in light of Kay's guilty plea.

In an unusual move, the judge said, 'It strikes me that it may not be in the interests of justice to pursue the other counts when the defendant has pleaded guilty to a substantive count like that.

'It is a serious charge that appears to address exactly what happened. Wouldn't it be better to accept it now rather than let this defendant get tangled up in a messy trial for the sake of some legal mumbo-jumbo?'

But prosecutor Annabel Darlow said the CPS was pushing ahead with all the charges because blood tests might shed some doubt on how Lynn died. Kay, who was accompanied at court by her family, was given conditional bail – the prosecution evidently didn't consider her a threat to the public.

Brown ordered the case to be tried by a High Court judge and set a provisional trial date for six months later, 12 January 2010.

Kay would never accept the accusation that she had attempted to kill Lynn. She knew with every fibre of her being that this was not so. Her life had been dedicated to her daughter, and having at last to accept that Lynn no longer wished to live had been devastating. Yet, as a mother who had always put her daughter's needs first, what right did she have to stand in her way and force her to live? Whose needs would she be serving then?

Feeling that it was only sensible to be prepared for the possibility that soon she might not be able to return to the home where she had raised and cared for her children, Kay began to pack up her house. Folding away Lynn's clothes was the hardest task of all. The beautiful dresses that were never worn, chosen together and talked about when they had sat and imagined a time that never came.

Lewes Crown Court, a Grade II listed building in the High Street of this elegant Sussex town, has seen many dramatic trials since its building was completed in 1812. Perhaps the most notorious is still the 1949 conviction of George John Haigh, the Acid Bath murderer, who dissolved the corpses of at least six of his female victims in acid as a means of escaping detection. But forensic evidence proved his guilt and he was hanged.

Half a century later, in 2001, Roy Whiting was found guilty of the murder of eight-year-old Sarah Payne, whom he had snatched from a cornfield in Sussex while out playing. Whiting was sentenced to life imprisonment for the crime, which had horrified the nation.

And it was here in this historic building that Kay Gilderdale's trial began on 12 January 2010.

Those called to jury duty for this trial were given the

option to stand down if they had strong feelings about euthanasia.

High Court judge Mr Justice Bean told potential jurors: 'If you have such strong views on the subject of assisted suicide one way or the other, if you feel you cannot give a true verdict on the evidence in this case and your name is one of those called today, say when you come forward and tell me about it.'

Of the first twelve names drawn randomly from the pool, one woman was released after speaking privately to the judge about personal circumstances which might affect her judgement in the case and a replacement was called up.

In the opening arguments delivered by the prosecution, the court was told how Kay, charged under her full name of Bridget Kathleen Gilderdale, helped end her daughter's life following Lynn's seventeen-year battle with illness by handing her a lethal dose of morphine and a cocktail of drugs.

Kay passed two syringes filled with large doses of morphine to Lynn, who injected the pain-relieving medicine herself in a suicide bid at the family home.

The prosecution went on to allege that when it became clear that the dosage was insufficient to meet Lynn's wish to die, her mother searched the house for tablets which she then crushed with a pestle and mortar and administered via a naso-gastric tube.

In the hours that followed, Kay, who the prosecution conceded was 'devoted' to her sick daughter, gave her three syringes of air through an intravenous catheter with the intention of causing air embolisms. Lynn died later that morning, 4 December 2008, at home in Stonegate.

Jurors at Lewes Crown Court were then told that Miss Gilderdale suffered from an 'unimaginably wretched' illness and had expressed a clear desire in the past to end her own life.

Prosecutor Sally Howes QC had had many years of experience in both prosecuting and defending high profile cases. She had frequently worked with cases that demanded expertise in medical, pathological and scientific evidence, and so it is not surprising that she instructed the jury of six men and six women that it was not their task to judge the 'motives or morals' of the defendant, or to choose where their sympathies lay.

It was a key strategy on behalf of the prosecution, who privately doubted that any member of the public listening to the evidence would believe that Kay acted out of self-interest. What Ms Howes wanted the jury to focus on was straightforward: did Kay Gilderdale's actions fall outside the law?

The charges that Kay faced were those of attempted murder, which she denied, and aiding and abetting suicide, which she admitted, between the second and the fifth of December 2008.

The jury was instructed that she could not be tried for murder as it was uncertain whether her daughter died from the overdose she gave to herself, or that given by her mother.

Ms Howes said: 'It is the prosecution's case that when Mrs Gilderdale realised that the two large doses of morphine that she provided to Lynn, that Lynn self-administered to try to end her life . . . instead of then realising that her daughter's suicide had gone horribly wrong, she then set about, over the next thirty hours, performing actions which were designed with no other intention other than terminating her daughter's life.

'The further morphine, the further cocktail of drugs, the injecting of air: all designed to terminate her daughter's life. It wasn't done to make her better, it was done to make sure she died.'

The prosecution, Ms Howes said, did not doubt that Mrs Gilderdale was a 'caring, loving and most devoted' mother: 'We don't doubt that Lynn Gilderdale suffered from a profound illness with a quality of life which was unimaginably wretched, and we do not dispute that Lynn had expressed a clear desire to end her life.

'The question for you to consider is what the defendant intended by her actions during those thirty fateful hours – the last thirty fateful hours of her daughter's life.

'The question for you to consider is whether the actions of Kay Gilderdale fell outside the law.'

The court heard how, more than a year before her death,

Lynn had accessed the website of Dignitas, and had also instructed a solicitor to draft a living will. They heard that the living will was countersigned by the family GP, Dr Jane Woodgate, who said she was satisfied that Lynn was of sound mental capacity at the time.

Ms Howes described how Lynn had at first suffered with panic attacks and spasms, and within four months was unable to move from the waist down and unable to sit up without losing consciousness. She became totally bedridden and lost her ability to swallow, which resulted in her having to be fed by a naso-gastric (nasal) tube.

Jurors heard how she communicated through sign language, which she developed with her parents who, although divorced, remained united in support of their daughter.

With her condition requiring numerous hospital admissions, Lynn was said to have grown to distrust the medical profession. She became heavily dependent on her mother and other carers.

Ms Howes said it was at about eight-thirty a.m. on 4 December 2008 that Lynn's father, Richard Gilderdale, telephoned Dr Woodgate's surgery to inform her that his daughter had died. Shortly afterwards, Dr Woodgate arrived at the Gilderdales' home where Kay told her the sequence of events that had led up to Lynn's death. She told the doctor that her daughter called out to her, saying she felt she had not administered enough morphine.

Kay had spoken to her daughter for about an hour, telling her it was 'not the right time' but Lynn insisted it was time for her 'to go'. She had said, 'I want the pain to go. I don't want to go on.'

At about three a.m. on 3 December, Kay gave her daughter two syringes of morphine containing 210 milligrams each, which Lynn administered herself through her Hickman line directly into her vein.

'At about six a.m. Kay felt that the morphine had not achieved Lynn's aim of killing herself and so Kay searched the house for tablets,' said Ms Howes. The tablets were crushed with a pestle and mortar and inserted into Lynn's naso-gastric tube.

Ms Howes continued her argument by telling the court that at about two a.m. on 4 December, Kay gave her two or three doses of morphine directly into the Hickman line and later gave her three syringes of air in the hope of stopping her heart with an air bubble.

Ms Howes said Kay telephoned the assisted suicide organisation, Exit, in the hope of gaining further advice, and then gave her daughter a further eight tablets. Lynn died at ten minutes past seven that morning. There were no signs of struggle and no suicide note was found, Ms Howes told jurors. When Kay was arrested on suspicion of murder, she said nothing.

A post-mortem examination carried out at the Conquest Hospital found that the cause of death was morphine toxicity (poisoning). Ms Howes said it was not possible to confirm from the blood sample the account given by Kay to Dr Woodgate about how many drugs had been administered.

Giving evidence, Dr Woodgate said Kay had explained she gave her daughter the drugs 'because she was frightened that Lynn would be brain damaged and not actually dead'.

Dr Woodgate said that Kay told her she had handed her daughter two syringes containing 210mg of morphine, which her daughter then administered herself. 'I understand Lynn went to sleep ... but then started to be very restless and wake up.' Kay told Dr Woodgate how she then gave her daughter a mixture of ground-up anti-depressants, tranquillisers and sleeping pills after contacting Exit, the right-to-die organisation, and then injected her with up to three syringes of air.

On the second day of the trial, it was the turn of Richard Gilderdale to take the stand. He told the court of his daughter's determination to rid herself of her suffering by ending her own life.

Richard Gilderdale sobbed in the witness box as he told the court that his daughter was determined to die after years of pain, telling him, 'My body is broken, Dad.'

He insisted that his ex-wife had done nothing but care for their daughter, who had grown to hate and fear hospitals after a 'catalogue' of bad experiences, including the alleged sexual assault. The former police sergeant said his ex-wife had selflessly helped their daughter kill herself and had not told him in order to protect him from the law.

Fiona Horlick, defending, said, 'You must realise now that she was protecting you from becoming involved.'

With tears in his eyes, he replied, 'Absolutely. She was doing what she had done for the last seventeen years – she was just devoted to Lynn.'

Describing the impact of their daughter's death, he said, 'We are never going to get over it. We are not just talking December 2008. The previous seventeen years and subsequent thirteen months of these proceedings have torn the family apart.'

He told the court he learnt that his daughter had died after he received a text message from his former wife saying, 'Please can you come now. Be careful. Don't rush.'

Jurors also heard from Lynn's carer and former neighbour, Julie Cheeseman, that 'she [Lynn] couldn't have got a better nurse than her own mum. She [Kay] was very devoted to her.'

When Lynn told Ms Cheeseman she had contacted Dignitas, Ms Cheeseman tried to talk her out of it. 'I told her that there is a light at the end of the tunnel, but I just don't think she wanted to be around," she said. "She just told me that she had had enough of her life and she wanted to die.'

Ms Cheeseman said Kay would often cut short planned trips away from looking after her daughter. She agreed with

Miss Horlick when she said that Kay's daughter was the most important aspect of her life, and that she never gave up hope for her.

The next day the jury heard that internet searches on how to commit suicide had been made on Kay's computer. In the hours leading up to Lynn's death, her mother trawled websites searching for methods on how to overdose on pills, and some of the search terms also related to morphine overdoses.

The searches were said to have been made by Kay over the course of the 'thirty fateful hours' leading up to Lynn's death.

The court was read a list of search phrases, websites and forums accessed on the computer in the hours before Lynn died. One of the items accessed related to news material about voluntary euthanasia campaigner Dr Philip Nitschke, dubbed 'Dr Death', and the 'suicide workshops' he was holding in the UK. One of the final searches before Lynn died was for an assisted suicide organisation.

That Kay played a significant role in Lynn's death was undeniable. That she loved her daughter was never questioned. But the prosecution was adamant that her actions fell outside the law. It was left to the jury to decide Kay's fate after the ten-day trial. It did not take them long.

The trial of Kay Gilderdale attracted massive media coverage. When the jury returned a verdict of not guilty, Kay was immediately besieged by family and friends, while the public gallery erupted in cheers. Kay then smiled and said, 'Thank you, thank you.'

Outside the court her son, Steve, spoke. With his mother and father alongside him, Steve Gilderdale said, 'We believe this not guilty verdict properly reflects the selfless actions my mother took on finding that Lynn had decided to take her own life, to make her daughter's final moments as peaceful and painless as possible.

'These actions exhibit the same qualities of dedication, love and care that Mum demonstrated throughout the seventeen years of Lynn's illness.

'I'm very proud of her and I hope she will be afforded the peace that she deserves to rebuild her life and finally grieve for her daughter.'

Speaking of the devotion he and his former wife showed to their daughter during her lifetime, Richard said, 'We nursed Lynn way past the line that ninety-nine per cent of members of the public would.'

That may well have been true, but it was Richard Gilderdale's words of love for his daughter and his faith in the actions of his former wife that resonated in every heart.

6

Acts of Mercy

The verdict on the case of Frances Inglis had been arrived at only five days before the jury in the Kay Gilderdale case had sat down to consider theirs.

It was very unusual that two high-profile cases involving mothers and their roles in the deaths of their children should be played out in the courts in the same week, and the intense publicity they generated served to underline the complex arguments and high emotions involved in ending the life of anyone with a serious or debilitating illness.

But no matter how much these two mothers, both women in their fifties who had dedicated themselves to their children, may have had in common, the issues surrounding Frances's case were very different from those of Kay's. Certainly, the nature of the revelations that came to light in the Inglis trial, made it even more dramatic than the Gilderdale trial.

Frances had been remanded in custody ahead of her trial. No application for bail was made at the hearing, perhaps less on the grounds that Mrs Inglis might abscond or commit further offences than by the fact that concerns were expressed over her state of mind and her health.

The trial was set to begin on 5 January 2010 at what is generally regarded as the most famous court in the world, the Central Criminal Court, or Old Bailey as it is universally known. It was expected to last three weeks.

Situated between St Paul's Cathedral and Holborn Circus, in the heart of the City of London, the court occupies a spot where trials have been taking place since mediaeval times. Known as the Old Bailey after the ancient fortified wall or 'bailey' that used to stand there, its most famous feature is the gold statue of a helmeted figure of Justice, standing guard atop the building's dome, holding a set of scales in her left hand and a raised sword in her right.

So often has the phrase 'justice is blind' been used, and so many images been seen of Justice with her eyes covered – many of them in cartoons or caricatures depicting an unseeing judicial system – that a great number of people assume, incorrectly, that the statue really is blindfolded.

Below the statue of Justice, and above the doors, an inscription carved in stone reads *Defend the children of the poor and punish the wrongdoer*. The words are taken from Psalm 72 of the Bible. Inside, on the court benches, are the Latin words *Domine, Dirige Nos*, translated as 'Lord, direct us' – though it is possible that those facing trial might think 'God, help us' would be more appropriate.

Among the countless thousands who have faced trial in this imposing building have been wife-murderer Dr Crippen; the former Liberal Party leader Jeremy Thorpe, who was acquitted of conspiracy to murder the ex-male-model Norman Scott; Peter Sutcliffe, the Yorkshire Ripper; the World War II traitor William Joyce, known as Lord Haw-Haw, and Ruth Ellis, the last woman to be hanged in Britain (for the murder of her lover). The notorious gangsters the Kray twins also stood in the Old Bailey dock, where Ronnie Kray told the judge at his 1968 trial for murder that, if he had not been required in court, he would 'probably have been having tea with Judy Garland'.

There were no such glamorous missed meetings pencilled in Frances Anne Inglis's diary on that first Tuesday in January, a bitterly cold day with snow in the air, when her trial began, and the story unfolded of Thomas Inglis's death and the events leading up to it.

As the proceedings opened with the case against her being presented to the jury by Miranda Moore QC, prosecuting, Frances – wearing a green cardigan, open-neck blouse and black trousers – sat listening in the dock, her head bowed.

This was, said Miss Moore, a 'tragic case', and gave an account of how Thomas had come to fall from an ambulance after a night out. The court heard how the then twenty-one-year-old required emergency surgery at Queen's Hospital. It was said that, despite remaining fully dependent on nursing care and having to be fed through a tube, Thomas began to make a steady improvement.

The upset that followed Tom's injury had affected all the members of the Inglis family. The extent of that suffering became clearer as more and more evidence was presented to the court.

Miss Moore said that Frances Inglis became 'obsessive', convinced that her son was in constant pain, and that two months later she made her first attempt to end his life. Lawyers for Frances, Miss Moore said, had written to the Crown Prosecution Service after she was charged with attempted murder, saying she admitted giving Tom heroin 'to kill him as an act of mercy', then, while out on bail, Frances began to consider what she should do next to end her son's life. Tom's death, when it came fourteen months later, was a 'meticulously planned operation', the court heard.

Frances Inglis, stated the prosecutor, had given her son a fatal overdose of heroin after gaining access to him at the Neuro Centre in Sawbridgeworth by using a false name. Once inside her son's room, she barricaded the door until staff who had been alerted managed to force their way in.

They restrained Frances in a bear hug while she shouted, 'Don't try to resuscitate him' and accused the staff of being 'stupid people' who didn't care about her son when he was alive. Miss Moore said, 'When she realised he was dead, she collapsed into a chair.' Asked how much heroin she had given him, Frances had replied, 'Ten little parcels – more than someone who takes heroin would take.'

Miss Moore's assessment of Frances's actions was stark: 'It is not a defence to murder or to attempted murder that a mother wants to put her son out of his misery, whether that misery is real or, as in this case, merely perceived.

'She thought he was suffering, that is why she did what she did. That is not a defence to murder. You are not entitled to terminate somebody's life in this way.'

The court heard that Frances had taken part in an online debate 'over the ethics of keeping her son alive', and that she had written on the website, 'I gave my son a heroin overdose to end his unimaginable suffering.'

Miss Moore acknowledged that Tom was wholly dependent on nursing care, transferred in and out of bed on a hoist, and fed via a tube, but she also emphasised that in the view of those responsible for treating him, making progress.

After Frances's first attempt on Tom's life, there had been a disagreement among experts about how badly what she did had affected her son's health and life expectancy, said Miss Moore; her actions could well have hindered any progress that might have been possible. She may well have shut the door on any likelihood of partial recovery.

When it came to how Frances had set out for the Centre in Hertfordshire, Miss Moore again emphasised that, 'This was a meticulously planned offence and she had made provision for what would happen to her and other people if she was arrested.'

When Tom's elder brother Alex took the stand, it was to much anticipation in the courtroom. Here was a son who had to give evidence for the prosecution about his mother's state of mind after Tom's accident. He said that Frances had become 'obsessive and negative' about the situation. On the second day of the trial, Alex told the jury how his brother's condition had driven his mother almost 'insane'. Tom had been left helpless and unable to speak and she believed he was being tortured by constant pain, the court heard.

Alex said that he and his father had initially been more hopeful than his mother about the chances of his brother's recovery. It had been suggested to the family, he added, that Tom could one day be 'walking, talking and running his own business. They told us Tom could get to that sort of level. I wanted to believe it at the time but I was never a hundred per cent.'

He said that his mother did not believe in the opinion of Tom's brain surgeon at Queen's Hospital, Mr Ragu Vindlacheruvu, that Thomas might make a recovery where he would regain his independence and be well enough to run his own business. Later, he himself grew more sceptical about these suggestions, and his mother thought them 'ridiculous'.

Eventually, he and his father began to discuss the 'probability' that Tom's life should be ended by obtaining a court order to allow his hydration and nutrition to be withdrawn. 'It was the only legal way it could happen, for Tom to die of hunger,' he said.

Sasha Wass QC, defending, asked Alex whether his mother had been left 'devastated' by the suggestion. He replied, 'It is horrific. I told her it is the only way that it could happen, for someone to die of thirst. It is sick.' He added that he had not directly asked her if she would consent but said he 'seriously doubted' that she would. His mother, he said, thought this approach 'horrific' and 'sick'.

Within days of the discussions, Tom was dead.

Alex told the court that his mother believed her son was in 'extreme pain' twenty-four hours a day. He said, 'She was constantly frantic and crying and just in a crazy state. You couldn't speak to her. She almost seemed to be insane. Her wish was that Tom would be dead, and at peace.

'She thought he was constantly in pain, so she could never relax. She could never go to sleep because she thought Tom's in pain, Tom's being tortured. That's the word she used.'

Alex also told the court that his mother believed Tom ought to have been left to die after his accident. 'She said that he shouldn't have been resuscitated, that he should have died naturally, that they shouldn't have been messing around with his brain to keep him alive.'

*

But when the trial entered its second week, the jury had the opportunity to hear crucial testimony from Thomas Inglis's surgeon.

Taking the stand, Mr Ragu Vindlacheruvu asserted that Tom could have gone on to 'make quite a favourable recovery'. He had cared for him at Queen's Hospital, Romford, and told the jury that Tom had shown 'little in the way of what seemed irrecoverable brain injuries'. In fact, he said, 'The early signs were about as good as we could have had at that stage.'

Mr Vindlacheruvu was asked by Miranda Moore QC how he would have described Mr Inglis's chances of recovery at the time:

'I will have said that it is possible that he may still die whilst an in-patient – and if no other complications arise he may go on to make quite a favourable recovery.

'Based on my personal experience of looking after young people with head injuries it was possible that he could end up independent, working, self-caring. I would emphasise that this was based upon my own personal experience of looking after head injuries – not simply reading miracle stories seen elsewhere.'

Hearing from a doctor who had years of experience working in the field of traumatic head injuries that it was possible Tom might have recovered was disturbing. And there was further alarming testimony given by Mr Vindlacheruvu. He told the jury that after Tom's subsequent cardiac arrest, his patient 'never recovered to what he was like . . . After September he was not showing the signs of improvement he had been showing.' This would prove to a crucial testimony.

The defence team produced other medical experts who stated that Mr Vindlacheruvu's opinion could be considered optimistic and also that it was possible to say that there was no real recordable change to Tom's responses on either side of Frances's attempt on his life but Mr Vindlacheruvu's testimony was enough to cast doubt over his mother's assertions about her son's condition.

On 13 January it was Frances Inglis's turn to give her version of events. She wept as she described how she wanted her son 'to go to Heaven rather than suffer Hell on earth'. She broke down in tears as she told the jury she believed the ordeal being suffered by her son was like being 'tortured'.

'We knew that he'd never be back to Tom,' she said. 'But if it would have been a quality of life that he enjoyed I would have been so happy for him and been with him and nursed him through it all if that's what he would have wanted. But if it was going to be a total horror story for him – I can't explain now how it was.'

She said every doctor she spoke to, apart from the consultant treating her son, had confirmed her worst fears.

'Tom has lost his life, didn't die, and would never be able to do anything himself,' she said. 'It would be like being buried alive and never being released, being tortured. I felt that he'd been kidnapped and was being tortured for no reason, for nothing other than, I don't know. It is just so unbearably cruel. It is so wrong, it is so wrong, it is so wrong to do that to somebody's brain.

'It is wrong to do it to my son, to see my son go through that – too much to bear, too much to bear.'

In hushed silence, the court listened as Frances spoke of her close and loving relationship with her son and of the awful moment she was told how he had suffered brain injuries after falling out of an ambulance in July 2007.

She said the family was told by a doctor that he would die unless he underwent an operation to remove part of his brain.

'I said to him no ... I understood it to be that they would keep him alive in terrible disability.

'I know Tom – no way would he have wanted to live totally dependent. I can remember saying I felt I would rather he go to heaven than to hell on earth. I know Tom would not want to live. He had lost his life.'

Nevertheless, the operation went ahead, the court heard, and a nurse who had lost her own son comforted her, Frances said.

'She said to me, "My son's in Heaven." I said I wish they'd let Tom go there too.' Frances added that she believed her son was kept alive because he had fallen out of an ambulance. She said if he died it would have 'looked very bad for them', adding: 'I know that the operation wasn't for Tom's benefit.' Frances had researched the outlook for her son's condition on the internet and had contacted an organisation called Headway that dealt with brain injuries.

As if the evidence she had given that day had not been tragic enough, there was even more anguish the next day when she continued to answer questions about the life and death of her son.

She told how two months after the accident she gave Tom an overdose that stopped his heart, how he was revived and she was arrested, and how and why she went back and injected him again, this time with the fatal dose of heroin, in November 2008.

'I felt he lost his life when he came out of the ambulance,' Frances told the court. 'I felt that I was helping, releasing him. I don't see it as killing or murder. The definition of murder is to take someone's life with malice in your heart.

'I did it with love in my heart, for Tom, so I don't see it as murder. I knew what I was doing was against the law. I don't know what name they would call it but I knew that the law would say it was wrong.

'I believed it would have been Tom's choice to have been allowed to die rather than have the intervention to keep him alive.'

She shook with sobs as she said, 'I had no choice, I had no choice. I would have chosen anything else, I would have done anything else. It is not that I wanted to do it, I had to.

I couldn't leave my son there. It is not an easy decision to make or something that anybody would want to do. I had no choice.'

Describing the first attempt in September 2007 she said, 'I had been on a nursing course so I had basic training about how to administer an injection . . . I got the heroin and I looked up on the internet how to use it and what the regular dose would be. Two grams, that would be a lethal dose.'

She went to his bedside with the heroin hidden in her handbag. She said she made notes of the times her son was being looked after to make sure she would not be disturbed as she injected him: 'I obviously wanted to do it properly.'

On two days she had been unable to find an opportunity to be alone with her son to administer the fatal dose. On the third occasion there was a staff shortage and she saw her chance.

'I was with Tom on my own,' she said. 'I held him, told him I loved him, told him everything was going to be fine, took the syringe, and I injected him in his thigh and his arm. Then he went to sleep. He was at peace. I stayed with him. Then he "died", he was at peace.'

After this effort to recall her first attempt to end Tom's life, Frances broke down and sobbed uncontrollably, but her testimony was not at an end. She had to go on to describe the horror she had felt at discovering that doctors had resuscitated her son after she left the hospital. It was like the doctors had 'put a knife in her,' she said. 'It was the cruellest thing they could do to Tom.'

This failed attempt to 'release' Tom made her all the more determined to succeed on another occasion. The jury had heard that there was a suggestion that her son's feeding might be withdrawn if it was decided it was no longer in his best interests to continue it. That would be a 'very very cruel, very very painful way' to die, Frances said. 'The only, only thing I could do was what I decided to do.'

She said she could think of nothing else but her son and his pain and the 'terror' she saw in his eyes – her son still had 'emotions, although he couldn't express them in words'.

On the morning that she went to Sawbridgeworth she laid out instructions at home for paying the bills and feeding the dog because she knew that she would be arrested. Then she gave an account of that last visit to her son.

'He was in bed. I told him that I loved him and I took the syringe and injected him in each thigh and in his arm and held him and told him I loved him, told him everything would be fine.

'I was very worried they were going to resuscitate him. I told them anything to keep them away from me. I didn't have HIV, obviously. I knew I had to help Tom. I couldn't relieve his suffering, I couldn't help him. I couldn't care for him. I asked myself what would Tom want. I asked myself what would I want. I would want someone to love me enough to help me and I knew I had to help him.'

Asked what had motivated her she said, 'Just totally, totally, utterly concerned for Tom. For Tom to live that living hell – I couldn't leave my child like that. I just couldn't do it, and I could think of nothing else.'

She had begun researching her son's condition on the internet within days of his accident, and she also told of how she begged staff at Queen's Hospital in Romford to give him relief for his 'terrible pain' and the 'look of sheer horror' on his face as he suffered fits of sweating and frothing at the mouth.

Frances, who said she used to visit her son twice a day, was asked by her barrister, Sasha Wass QC, about the 'encouraging' prognosis described by consultant surgeon Mr Vindlacheruvu. She replied: '[He had suggested] that Tom might be running his own business, walking, talking, independent, totally opposed to what everyone else had said and what I had seen with my own eyes.

'All I saw was horror, pain and tragedy. I knew I had to help him. I asked myself what Tom would want. He wouldn't have wanted to live like this. That's why I thought heroin – a painless, peaceful death.'

She told how she tried unsuccessfully to obtain the drug from a neighbour before looking elsewhere. 'I'd go to places where I thought maybe deals were made, like Barking station and outside the job centre. I tried to find out where the needle exchange places were,' she told the court.

Eventually she obtained needles and syringes from the hospital and learnt from the internet that two grams of heroin would be a 'lethal dose'. It was never revealed exactly where or from whom she had bought the heroin or if they had any idea what Frances had intended to do. Whoever sold Frances the drug did not question why a woman in her fifties was buying two grams of the narcotic, not an insubstantial amount.

Once Frances learnt that the only legal way for Tom to die would be via an application to the High Court to withdraw his feeding, she was horrified. These applications are something that generally can only be done after the patient has been in a persistent vegetative state for twelve months. Although her son had not been so classified, the possibility of such an application had been raised in a medical report about him. Frances said, 'I could not bear the thought of Thomas dying of thirst and hunger. To die slowly like that would be horrible.'

Two weeks after the trial had begun, the jury heard the customary closing speeches from both the prosecution and defence counsels.

Sasha Wass QC for the defence said that Tom's injuries had left him in what Frances saw as a living hell. He was imprisoned in a useless body, unable to communicate, unable to experience any pleasure or enjoyment of life in the real sense.

'She saw the pain and the fear and the terror in his eyes. You imagine seeing the person you love most in the world in that condition,' Miss Wass said. 'In her view she had not killed him but saved him from an agonised existence. She gave Tom the peace that he had been denied.'

Miranda Moore QC for the State acknowledged that '. . . it would be a hard-hearted person who didn't have sympathy for her position,' but, she said, the case must not be decided on emotion and sympathy; people must not be permitted to take the law into their own hands.

In this assertion, Miss Moore would be echoed a week later by Sally Howes QC during Kay Gilderdale's trial. But Miss Moore was able to make clear distinctions between the cases of Frances and Kay – the wishes of the deceased: 'It is not for one person to decide what should happen, no matter how pure their motives. The law in this country has to be – and is – very clear.'

It was not suggested that Inglis was a bad mother, said Miss Moore, but that she had convinced herself that she alone knew what was best for her son.

'We are not saying she had evil intentions. We are just saying she had illegal ones, misguided ones. It is a tragic case, but it is not a defence to murder to end someone's life to put them out of their misery.'

The seven-man, five-woman jury returned its verdict after deliberating for six hours and twenty-one minutes. By a majority of ten to two they returned a verdict of guilty on both charges – murder and attempted murder. Their decision was greeted with cries of 'Shame on you' from the public gallery. The Inglis family were very obviously upset.

Frances Inglis hung her head in silence as the verdict was announced.

Mr Justice Barker had told the jury no-one had the 'unfettered right' to take the law into their own hands; he thanked them, and also told them that 'You could not have had a more difficult case'.

Then, addressing Frances, Judge Barker said, 'You were a devoted mother, highly regarded for your work in the community . . . [But] However we look at all this, this was a calculated and consistent course of criminal conduct. This is a highly unusual and very sad case. I accept that his life and yours were changed on July 7th.

'What you did was to take upon yourself what you thought your son's wishes would have been, to relieve him from what you described as a living hell.

'But you cannot take the law into your own hands and you cannot take away life, however compelling you think the reason.'

'This was not an act of legal altruism,' the judge said, 'although we can all understand the emotion and the unhappiness that you were experiencing. The fact is that you knew that you intended to do a terrible thing. You knew you were breaking society's conventions, you knew you were breaking the law, and you knew the consequences.'

He imposed a minimum jail term of nine years, a term allowed under sentencing guidelines because of the 'mercy killing' nature of the case.

Having already served 423 days on remand, which would be deducted from her sentence, Frances would be eligible for parole in seven and a half years.

It is worth noting at this stage that judges, when considering how long a murderer should serve in jail, work out their minimum recommendation (in all but the most horrific cases) from a starting point of fifteen years.

They then add or subtract years, depending on the seriousness of the killing. Mitigating factors which will reduce the punishment include 'a belief by the offender that the murder was an act of mercy'.

A former Lord Chief Justice, Lord Woolf, set guidelines in 2002 which put the proper minimum jail term for a murderer in a mercy killing at eight or nine years. However, judges have since given lower sentences such as when, in 2007, Mr Justice Silber tried fifty-eight-year-old former accountant Frank Lund at Liverpool Crown Court for the killing of his wife Patricia. The jury found Mr Lund guilty of murder for suffocating his wife with a plastic bag and a pillow to free her from the pain of illness.

The judge, who said Mr Lund had acted at his wife's request and from a misguided sense of loyalty, set a minimum term of three years.

It was with knowledge of such compassionate judgements as that, that Frances's son Alex wanted a review of the law for people in his mother's position who kill as an 'act of mercy'.

In Frances's case, the judge's remarks and his sentence were not to be the end of the matter.

Far from it.

7

Aftershock

The two very different outcomes of the Inglis and Gilderdale trials prompted much comment, a good deal of it focusing on the key question of whether it can ever be right to take the life of someone you love if they are unable to act for themselves, or express their own wish to die.

For Kay, it had been a much simpler (if not any the less painful) set of circumstances. That Lynn no longer wished to continue her struggle against her illness was entirely clear. She wrote with heartbreaking clarity about the harsh reality of her limited and painful life, and bravely about her decision to end it. Thomas Inglis left no such legacy. He was unable to communicate his needs, something that pained his mother greatly, but significantly, neither could he relay his wishes about whether he preferred to live or die.

Frances had acted on instinct, on her knowledge of her son's character and a close understanding of how she believed he would have viewed his predicament before the accident. She fervently believed that he would have refused to live in such a truncated and distressing state. But, crucially, it was *her* belief – not Tom's clear and unambiguous insistence that he no longer wished to live after the accident.

The medical community could not give the Inglis family any guarantee that Tom would one day reclaim his life, but neither did his surgeon write off his patient's chances of regaining a functioning independence.

Frances first decided to try to end Tom's life only ten days after his hospitalisation, even if she didn't carry out an attempt until some weeks later. She subsequently admitted to detectives that she was highly distraught, and when she wrote about her fears that Tom was tortured by pain she said, 'I was sort of off my head really.' Beset by grief and a terrible fear that Tom was suffering, it can be argued that her judgement was compromised.

Grief, confusion and fear of events slipping further out of control and harming her son yet more hint at the turmoil that raged in Frances. The thought of Tom suffering and so horribly reduced was unbearable to Frances and some questioned if this distress – and an unconscious desire to end it – had played a part in her actions. The weight of guilt and grief packed into one simple statement reveals that distress: *I couldn't help him. I couldn't care for him.*

No one doubted that Frances loved her son, but the jury had arrived at the legally correct decision that she had acted unlawfully.

Frances's family rallied to her defence. Alex – who, let it

be remembered, had appeared as a prosecution witness – gave the following statement:

'I want to say that all of the family, and Tom's girlfriend, support my mum a hundred per cent. All of those who loved and were close to Tom have never seen this as murder, but as a loving and courageous act. Why is my mum the only person who has been called to answer for her actions which were done out of love for her son?

'What this case and a number of others have exposed is a need for a complete rethink of existing laws in regard to people that have been, and will be, in the same position as Tom.

'How can it be legal to withhold food and water, which means a slow and painful death, yet illegal to end all suffering in a quick, calm and loving way?

'It's cruel and illogical. The law simply isn't keeping pace with modern medicine and aggressive surgery, which is wrong as it leaves too many people in such tragic and painful existences.

'We have a duty of care to them and should not allow this situation to continue. It should not be left to a wife, mother, father, sister or brother to have to end their suffering, and then be convicted of murder.'

The family also said there were still questions which needed answering about how Thomas fell from the ambulance.

Describing his mother's pain, Alex had said, 'She was

constantly frantic and crying and just in a crazy state.'
Now, a few days after sentence was passed on his mother,
Alex said, 'She is OK. For the first time she's calm and said
she would rather be in prison than seeing Tom suffering and
existing in a way she knows he would have hated. I spoke
to her today and she was just saying thanks for all the
support.

'But we're devastated she's being punished for ending his
life humanely. Tom was always really, really independent.
He always said don't make a fuss. Being in that state, he
would have hated it.'

All of the family and all who loved Tom had been forced
to ask themselves difficult questions about the path Frances
had taken and Alex was no exception. He said, 'At first I
clung to the possibility of Tom getting better. Mum kept
saying we can't leave him like this. She couldn't bear the
thought of him suffering. At the beginning, although we
couldn't communicate with him, Tom had this embarrassed
look about him. I can't describe it but I could just tell
because he's my brother.

'He would have hated other people tending to him,
seeing him undressed and washing him, that would've been
his idea of hell. Other times he would grimace in pain and
it was horrible to watch. It tortured my mum and she was
completely different to how she had been before.

'She'd be with him as much as she could, giving him
head massages and talking to him. She was only ever calm

with him because she didn't want him to see how upset she was.

'Other times she was constantly devastated. When Tom was given the first overdose, at first I was angry with Mum because I thought maybe he could get better. But we were clutching at straws. After about two months I realised she was right.

'She isn't a murderer. We could have got permission to withhold Tom's food and water so he starved to death which is an evil, cowardly way to end someone's life. Our family would not have allowed it.'

Love can inspire emotions so profound that any act, even one of extremes, might be contemplated if it means releasing a loved one from pain. Alex admitted, 'I was actually considering killing him myself. I was planning a trip to France and once I got back I was going to end his life. My mum didn't come to this decision lightly. She's devastated her son's gone, but knows he isn't suffering any more.'

Passions ran high. Every reader of a newspaper could imagine themselves trapped in the invidious position of having to decide what a loved one rendered mute through injury or illness would wish.

Frances Inglis had even questioned whether anyone in her life loved her enough to help her end it if she were to become a wasted shell.

Knowing that Frances faced a life sentence became even

more unpalatable when other prison sentences handed down in the same week were examined.

Mary Butres was sent to jail for seven and a half years, the day after Frances was sentenced. She was responsible for the deaths of two young people as a result of driving her Jaguar XJ8 at 113mph while intoxicated, and in bad weather.

To the families of the victims, Mary Butres committed an act of devastating negligence – as well as a criminal offence – but the law, as it stands, views premeditated murder as the greater offence.

In most cases the law's approach is a rational one. Unlike a death, however tragic, that results from an accident, in almost all instances, death resulting from a planned murder is morally repellent. Thus the judge in Frances's case underlined the 'calculated' nature of her attempts to take Tom's life which, ordinarily, would in itself justify a life sentence.

However, what this case and others like it exposed is that premeditated murder can take place without malice. The *mens rea*, or guilty mind, comes in many complex guises. Yes, Frances was intent on ending her son's life, but the questions of 'want' or 'personal gain' were far from clear cut.

It is difficult to see how a set of hard and fast rules can apply equally to each and every case, yet that is what we demand from the law. At its most favourable, the organic nature of the British legal system does allow for a nuance in interpretation of the law on a case-by-case basis. That was evident some years earlier, during the trial of Heather Pratten.

In 2000 Heather Pratten, then sixty-three, was tried at the Old Bailey for aiding and abetting the suicide of her son. At the conclusion of the trial, she stood in the dock, fighting back the tears when the judge said to her, 'Your story is one that would move the hardest of hearts.'

During the court proceedings, people in the public gallery had openly wept as the heart-rending tragedy of how Heather had helped her disease-stricken son Nigel to kill himself, was revealed in detail.

The court heard how Nigel had chosen the day of his forty-second birthday to end his suffering once and for all, and had made his mother promise that she would not let him leave his flat alive.

On that day, she arranged a row of birthday cards by his bed, and mother and son celebrated with a special lunch before she helped him to load a syringe and inject a heroin overdose into his arm. He also swallowed some of the drug dissolved in a spoon.

They sang 'Happy Birthday' together, and then Heather hugged him and held him in her arms while he drifted into unconsciousness. When it was clear that he was in a deep coma, she pressed a pillow over his face to smother his last gasps.

It was the hereditary brain illness Huntington's Disease which had affected Nigel and devastated Heather's family.

Her first husband had died after enduring the crippling condition for a decade and, at the time, another of her sons (she had had five children) was also afflicted with the disease.

The court heard that during hospitalisation Nigel expressed to a number of medical personnel, as well as to his family, his desire to return to his home and die, and he talked to those people about a number of ways of committing suicide.

Heather had taken her son from hospital to his home in Plaistow, East London where, the court heard, 'Once inside the flat he produced a foil wrap. He asked her to unwrap it. He told her then he was not going to return to the hospital and she must promise not to let him leave the flat alive. She tried to persuade him not to commit suicide but he was adamant.'

Thirty minutes after Nigel stopped breathing, Heather called an ambulance, telling the operator her son was dead.

Two syringes were found in the flat, along with a signed suicide note from Nigel, which read 'I am suffering and want to die.'

Heather's defence counsel addressed the court, saying, 'What has happened has had a very profound effect on her. She has endured suffering on behalf of the people she cared for and loved . . . Allow her to keep her liberty,' he pleaded.

Heather admitted aiding and abetting Nigel's suicide, but Judge Graham Boal freed her with a conditional discharge.

A decade before the Frances Inglis trial, Judge Boal expressed the view that Heather Pratten had suffered enough. He told her she was a 'good, caring and brave woman', and went on to say, 'I do not want to prolong your agony a moment longer than is absolutely necessary. Human life is precious – many regard it as sacred. Only in the rarest and most exceptional cases can those who contribute to the death of another be sentenced to anything other than imprisonment. Your case is exceptional.'

When Mrs Pratten left the Old Bailey a free woman, she said, 'I have just one thing I want to say and that is I have always believed in British justice, and today I was proved right.'

She later added, 'My son saw no reason to suffer the final years of his terrible disease and, because I would not leave him to die alone, it caused more suffering for our family when I was on bail for murder and finally pleaded guilty to aiding and abetting a suicide. I was forced to be alone, with no support, because of our outdated attitudes towards those who are capable of making decisions for themselves.'

Significantly, she also said, 'When it was all over, the only feeling I had was relief: he'd got what he desperately wanted. I would have loved to have been able to ask the medical profession for help. But I've never felt guilty about it, I've never regretted it, because I just know it was the right thing for him.'

*

Heather Pratten's involvement in her son's death clearly had more similarities to Kay Gilderdale's role in the death of Lynn. Nonetheless, ten years after her own ordeal, Mrs Pratten spoke out about the Frances Inglis case.

After Frances was sentenced, Mrs Pratten said that judges should have more discretion. 'I am not saying people should not be brought to account, but we need different terminology so that murder charges are not brought in such cases.

'Frances Inglis clearly isn't a murderer. She isn't a threat to the public and should not have been charged, let alone jailed. My situation was different because Nigel had told everyone about his desire to die. He had watched his father die from the illness and didn't want to go through the same thing. My other son also died from Huntington's and in the end couldn't swallow. He starved to death over ten days.

'Though Tom wasn't in a position to express a wish to die, I'm sure he was very close to his mother like I was to Nigel. It just had to end, which is why I picked up a pillow and put it over his face. I did it for love. What Frances did was out of love.'

Others also spoke out too to say that they understood what Frances had faced during her months of anguish. Forty-seven-year-old Nicky Dallady from Loughton, Essex, a multiple sclerosis sufferer for twenty-six years, had been diagnosed with the disease when she was twenty-one. She too wanted the right to end her life. 'I admire what Frances did,' she said. 'It takes a great amount of guts and it would be the last thing a mother would want to do to her son. You would die for your children and do anything to protect them.

'I agree with what she did. It was the right thing to do. I've had MS for twenty-six years. I rely on my husband for everything. To me, that's not a dignified life. My condition will never improve, it will only get worse.

'When I feel like I cannot go on any more, I would like to be able to die in this country. A lot is spoken of human rights, but what about my right to die with dignity?'

But not everyone offered unqualified support for Frances's actions. An opposing view came from former England Under-21 rugby player, Matt Hampson, then twenty-four, from Skeffington, Leicestershire, who had been paralysed from the neck down after breaking his neck in a scrum five years earlier.

'I never considered ending my life. I was healthy, it was just my spine that was knackered. I don't know why this mother did what she did, and I don't want to judge her. Everyone makes their own choices, and I decided to get busy living.

'Of course I had bleak times when I thought about everything I missed doing, everything I could do before, and I wondered if I would ever enjoy life again in the state

I was in. I had always been fiercely independent. Now, I couldn't even lift a drink to my lips.

'I'm a young guy and I didn't know if I would find another girlfriend, have sex again, get married, become a dad. I still don't, but I choose not to dwell. I've always been an upbeat person. I always try to look at what I can do, not what I can't.

'Most importantly, I couldn't have done it without the love and support of my family and friends.'

As well as individuals, organisations found themselves on opposing sides of the arguments. Dignity in Dying said they felt it 'inappropriate' for Frances to be tried for murder. Its chief executive, Sarah Wootton, said:

'We absolutely don't condone breaking the law, despite it being clear that Mrs Inglis was motivated by love and compassion. We are calling for the Government to revisit the Law Commission's 2006 report which found that a review was necessary into the way these cases are tried and whether there should be a specific defence of mercy killing [...] I don't think Frances Inglis did the right thing, but she was motivated by love and it's not helpful that she's been incarcerated. She's not a danger to society and putting her in prison won't achieve anything. But she was tried under murder law which doesn't have any discretion around mercy.

'This case acts as a sad reminder that we should all make our treatment wishes known to loved ones, and to our doctors, through an Advance Decision. Advance Decisions are legally binding documents which, if valid and applicable, must be respected. Had Tom Inglis had an Advance Decision stating that he refused life-sustaining treatment in the situation he found himself in, the doctors would have had to respect that refusal of treatment.

'Mrs Inglis's perception of Tom's condition was that there was no hope for his recovery, perhaps due to a lack of communication between health professionals and Tom's family. Given advances in medicine and changes to the law, the General Medical Council is in the process of creating guidelines for health professionals on end-of-life treatment and decision-making.

'We hope this will minimise discrepancies in care, treatment and information provision, and help to support health professionals to provide the best possible care and patient-centred choice at the end of life, for the benefit of both patients and their loved ones. Dignity in Dying looks forward to the publication of this guidance and hopes it will improve end-of-life care across the board.

'As with the abolition of slavery, the legalisation of abortion, and the decriminalisation of suicide, society faces an ethical and political issue in which pressure for change meets resistance. Like those we follow, change will come,' Ms Wootton concluded.

*

Dignity in Dying has set out, in its ten-point charter, its aims which they believe to be 'essential if people are to gain comfort, and peace of mind in the knowledge that they will be able to have a dignified death'. It is instructive at this stage to look closely at these aims:

1 Everyone should have the opportunity to create an End-of-Life Care Plan setting out their needs and wishes for the end of life, and should have access to good advice services to inform their choices.

2 Health professionals should have a duty to carefully consider people's wishes as set out in their End-of-Life Care Plan, such as their preferred place of care at the end of life.

3 Government should promote awareness of Advance Decisions so that everyone knows that they have a legal right to refuse treatment.

4 Advance Decisions must be recorded in a central National Health register so that health professionals can take them into account in treatment.

5 Building on the principles of choice and control at the end of life, Parliament must give terminally ill, mentally competent people the right to have an assisted death.

6 More resources should be made available for palliative care – Government must deliver on its manifesto commitment to double funding for palliative

care and all political parties should pledge to match this investment.

7 Decision makers should end the postcode lottery in accessing palliative care services by providing a consistent and transparent system for commissioning services.

8 Carers of terminally ill people should receive more support, with a Carers' Benefit introduced for all those providing thirty-five or more hours of care per week regardless of age; legal protection against employment discrimination for carrying out such a role; and better access to palliative care.

9 Health and social care professionals should have access to training on end-of-life issues, including offering emotional, psychological and spiritual support to patients; communication skills and high-quality bereavement skills.

10 Bereaved people should have easy access to advice services offering first-point-of-call assistance to other support such as legal and financial advice, and referral to counselling services, as appropriate.

But this is not the only campaign group focusing on the issues that surround assisted suicide. Care Not Killing is an organisation that describes itself as 'a UK-based alliance of individuals and organisations which brings together disability and human rights organisations, healthcare and palliative care groups, and faith-based organisations, with the aims of promoting more and better palliative care; ensuring that existing laws against euthanasia and assisted suicide are not weakened or repealed during the lifetime of the current Parliament, and influencing the balance of public opinion further against any weakening of the law.'

Care Not Killing aims to 'attract the broadest support among the very many in the medical profession and allied health services and in society at large who are opposed to euthanasia. It appeals to those of all faiths and none by adducing arguments based on reason alone, by avoiding any appeals to extremism, and by drawing on and developing a well-researched evidence base.' Its aims include:

1 Providing simple, compelling and clear campaigning under the slogan 'Care Not Killing' with supporting evidence to marshal support against Bills to legalise euthanasia or assisted suicide during the lifetime of the next Parliament;

2 Developing a network of expert spokespeople from core group member organisations and producing powerful advocacy in the media against euthanasia;

3 Funding opinion polls and supporting research where needed to increase support;

4 Monitoring developments in the courts;

5 Seeking to build up and mobilise mass political

support to be deployed with maximum impact on the parliamentary process as and when necessary;

6 To campaign positively for increased provision of better palliative care, including more funding for hospices and better residential care for the infirm elderly and for the dying, recognising that the fear of dying alone and in pain is a powerful driver of the pro-euthanasia movement.

The group clearly feared a rollback in legislation to such an extent that organised opposition was necessary.

Dr Peter Saunders, director of Care Not Killing, said the current law on assisted suicide and mercy killing acted as a powerful deterrent to protect vulnerable people from exploitation and abuse. He said:

'Many cases of financial, physical or emotional abuse occur within the context of so-called loving families. The law is there to protect carers from being subtly coerced into helping loved ones kill themselves, and also to protect vulnerable, sick or disabled people from succumbing to pressure, real or imagined, to end their lives so as not to be a burden to others.

'If we remove or lessen the penalty for so-called "mercy killing" we will leave vulnerable people without adequate legal protection and also contribute to a mindset that the lives of sick or disabled people are somehow less worth living.

'Both of these would be tremendously damaging to society. It is therefore extremely important that the current law, which holds tough penalties in reserve but gives discretion for judges to show leniency in hard cases, is upheld.'

And, commenting directly on the Frances Inglis trial, Dr Saunders said, 'This is a harrowing case which evokes strong emotions – but it is right that the law has been upheld. If judges failed in their duty to prosecute in hard cases like this it would undermine the deterrent effect of the law and would be a recipe for the abuse of many elderly and disabled people whose lives would inevitably be placed at risk.

'Even desperate relatives must never be allowed to take the law into their own hands. A change in the law to allow euthanasia or assisted suicide is dangerous because vulnerable people would inevitably feel under pressure to end their lives. It is unnecessary because compassionate alternatives exist.

'And it is just plain wrong as it is contrary to all historic codes of medical ethics. We embark on such a path at our peril.'

The law has to protect the vulnerable. It has to protect those who cannot defend themselves and it has to uphold the rights of those with a different quality of life from the well and able-bodied.

This is more than a rarefied question of ethics.

When Lord Falconer, the former Lord Chancellor, led the debate in the House of Lords and argued that the laws surrounding assisted suicide should be relaxed, it seemed that his reasoning would win the day. However, when Baroness Campbell of Surbiton began to speak, the tide began to turn. In measured tones, Baroness Campbell stated her views on the notion of a change in the current law. Not only those present in the House, but all those who witnessed her speech on television or read a summary of her arguments in press reports, were given cause to think again.

Baroness Campbell was born with spinal muscular atrophy, a degenerative disease that has robbed her of mobility and causes her to be frequently hospitalised with severe respiratory illnesses. On one occasion, barely able to breathe and unable to speak or swallow she heard doctors discussing her prognosis. They were deciding that it would be in her best interests to place 'Do Not Resuscitate' on her case notes.

Unable to speak for herself and fast losing consciousness, it was a terrifying experience. It was only the timely intervention of her husband, who insisted that the team do all they could to improve her condition, that saved the day.

This traumatic incident provided Baroness Campbell with a key insight. 'I know those doctors were trying to be kind, wanting to do what they thought was best for me, to ease my suffering by ending my life,' she said. 'But it wasn't what I wanted. And in my heart I knew that because these doctors didn't know me they would make assumptions. Assumptions that were utterly wrong.'

Our gauge of what is 'bearable' or of what is a 'life worth living' is necessarily a subjective one. Baroness Campbell knew that the doctors surrounding her had the best intentions, but when a patient – disabled through accident or a degenerative illness – is unable to speak, who should speak for them? Is it a 'natural' right of a spouse or a family member to decide? Is it fair or can it ever be right for doctors to bear the responsibility for 'end of life' decisions?

In an ideal world, of course, each of us would have an End-of-Life Care Plan, setting out our needs and wishes just as Dignity in Dying suggest. But, as with donor cards, each of us has good intentions but that does not always mean that we make the arrangements necessary for our wishes to be set out in advance. The irony is that death is the only outcome that is certain in life and yet, in our hundreds of thousands, we delay writing of wills, die intestate, and hope that our deaths will be pain-free, swift and uncomplicated.

For those who are struck down with terminal or degenerative illness, opportunity exists for them to set out their wishes. And it is these individuals who are challenging and changing the legal arguments and the moral landscape.

When Debbie Purdy, who has multiple sclerosis, won the right to decide to end her life if her suffering becomes too much to bear, public opinion backed her demand. The majority also understood her fight to establish exactly what would happen to her husband should she ask for his help in assisting her to die. Would he face a murder charge?

It was a groundbreaking case. Ms Purdy's lawyers demanded to know how the Suicide Act of 1961 would be enforced if, for example, her husband Omar Puente accompanied her to Switzerland to die. Debbie stressed that should her husband be placed at risk of prosecution, she would travel unassisted to the Dignitas clinic. Such a decision, and the journey itself would, however, have to be made while she was still physically capable of travelling unaccompanied – in other words, sooner than she would choose, or might actually be necessary, to end her life – if Omar was to remain within the law and safe from prosecution.

In February 2010, Ms Purdy learnt that, according to new guidelines set out by the Director of Public Prosecutions, Omar, if proven to have acted purely from motives of compassion, would not be pursued by the law. However, the DPP, Keir Starmer QC, was at pains to stress that 'The policy does not change the law on assisted suicide. It does not open the door for euthanasia.'

But for Debbie Purdy, this was a big step forward in protecting the choice of an individual and his or her family members. After the ruling, she said, 'The current guidelines are enough to give me my life back and to know that I can carry on living and don't have to worry about making a decision now.'

The overwhelming majority of the public backed Ms Purdy's desire for clarity and supported what appeared to be her basic human right to choose to end her life on her own terms.

But it does seem that the courage of our convictions starts to waver when we are asked if it is right to help someone to die if their condition is incurable but not fatal. An opinion poll for the BBC showed that a large majority – seventy-five per cent – of those polled, supported the right to die for those enduring a terminal illness. However, that support fell to only forty-eight per cent if the condition were not fatal, while forty-nine per cent said that they were actually opposed to assisted suicide in such cases.

Baroness Campbell's voice remains an essential one when such questions are pondered. Of Debbie Purdy's legal campaign, she has said, 'I would defend to the end her right to that opinion. But with rights come responsibilities. And I want to make heard the voice of an equally disabled woman who holds a wholly opposing view. You have to fight like with like.'

Doctors are frequently placed in a difficult dilemma. The Royal College of Physicians has warned that a relaxation of the law surrounding assisted death could mean that doctors are pressured by loved ones into speculating how long a patient has to live, thus escaping prosecution by claiming that the patient was terminally ill.

The arguments are ongoing. Nobody is confident or

satisfied that a simple set of legal rulings can create clarity, or serve the complex ethics and varying circumstances surrounding the right to die. Meanwhile, somewhere out there is always a family who will have to face a new and dreadful tragedy: the slow, painful and cruel decline – or the sudden and catastrophic end – of the functioning of a life they cherish.

And such a family, as matters stand, will be left to confront the same terrible questions that tormented Kay Gilderdale and Frances Inglis.

Eight

Somebody's Mother, Somebody's Son

—

Other stories need to be told of other families; families who found themselves the focus of a criminal investigation at a time that could not have been harder to bear.

This was the fate that befell Julie and Mark James, and as events unfolded their case become one that revealed crucial aspects about both Dignitas, the clinic that has come to dominate accounts of arranged suicides, and the dilemmas facing the Crown Prosecution Service.

Julie and Mark James's son Daniel was a young rugby player with the possibility of a bright future in the game. A talented forward for Nuneaton Rugby Club, he seemed destined for a professional career in Rugby Union. Having played for England at under-16 level, he moved on to play for Loughborough University, where he was an undergraduate engineering student.

In March 1967, hooker Daniel helped England Students beat a French side in a match in Oxford. Four days later, he was involved in a training accident: during a special training session he was attending for forwards, Daniel was practising a scrum when the rest of the pack came crashing down on him. For hookers to find themselves at the bottom of a pack is not unusual, but what happened to Daniel turned out to have terrible consequences.

The weight of the players on top of him dislocated the vertebrae in Daniel's neck, trapping his spinal cord and causing instant paralysis from the chest down.

In the following weeks, Daniel underwent several operations and then spent eight months in rehabilitation, including a period at Stoke Mandeville hospital, before returning home. Despite the care and expertise brought to bear in his case, the only movement the now paralysed former Royal Worcester School pupil had managed to regain was limited use of his fingers.

Daniel's father Mark, who had been Worcester's first XV hooker for several years, had to listen as his son described his body as a 'prison'. Daniel told Mark that he lived in 'fear and loathing' of his daily life, of the humiliations he endured in order to keep his body functioning. His parents not only had to come to terms with the fact that their son as they knew him was now lost to them, but had to cope with Daniel's repeated attempts to kill himself.

On 12 September 2008, Daniel James's life ended at a Dignitas clinic in Switzerland. He was just twenty-three, and was believed to be the youngest Briton ever to have gone abroad to commit suicide.

Nuneaton Rugby Football Club released a brief statement on their website:

> Following the tragic injury sustained by Dan James at a training session in March 2007, it is with great sadness that we have to report Dan passed away peacefully on Friday, 12 September.
>
> Our sympathies now lie with his family and we would ask that the family's privacy is honoured at this very difficult time for them.

His funeral took place in the UK on 1 October, and the news of the circumstances of his death became known in the middle of that month. Once the facts were public knowledge, his parents found that not only did they have to defend their son's decision to die, but that they were now subject to a police inquiry in connection with the inquest held over their son's death.

Mr and Mrs James, from Sinton Green, Worcester, issued a statement saying that Daniel was an intelligent young man of sound mind who was not willing to live what he felt was a second-class existence. They said their son had tried several times to kill himself before he got his wish to die. As Mark and Julie James expressed it:

'His death was an extremely sad loss for his family, friends and all those that care for him, but no doubt a welcome relief from the prison he felt his body had become and the day-to-day fear and loathing of his living existence, as a result of which he took his own life.

'This is the last way that the family wanted Dan's life to end but he was, as those who knew him are aware, an intelligent, strong-willed and, some say, determined young man.

'The family suffered considerably over the last few months and do wish to be left in peace to allow them to grieve appropriately.'

Daniel's parents said their son had never come to terms with his extreme physical incapacity: 'Over the last six months he constantly expressed his wish to die and was determined to achieve this in some way.' A spinal research fund created by family and friends in his memory had already raised almost £25,000.

Keith Howells, president of Nuneaton Rugby Football Club said of Daniel, 'He was a great player. One memory I've got is when we came back from winning a match away Dan was singing karaoke on the coach with a stupid hat on. That was the character of Dan. A great player and a great loss.'

Alan Buzza, director of rugby at Loughborough, said Dan was 'a tough boy, he had attitude, and was a good athlete and handler whose constructiveness with the ball also made him a good Sevens player. He was a big character – one of his nicknames was Cowboy – and he was a guy who lived life to the full and threw himself into everything wholeheartedly.'

After the accident, his mother, Julie, had told a local newspaper, 'It was so sudden. We had no build-up to it, it just happened. We got a phone call saying Dan had a bit of a knock at rugby. That was it.'

Before Dan's death, his uncle, Mark Roebuck, who started the Dan James Trust that raised the money for spinal research, paid tribute to his nephew: 'On Monday March 12th Dan was just like thousands of twenty-three-year-olds, full of life, hope, excitement and dreams. His life at university was full, active and successful, surrounded by fantastic mates, with the promise of employment in construction management if his rugby career did not continue to blossom.

'Whatever he chose to do, he would have done it with his usual good humour and lovely nature that have made him the lovable young man that he has grown into. He truly was on the threshold of life and he lived his life to the full and embraced every opportunity that came his way.'

Daniel had dislocated his C6/C7 vertebrae, trapping his spinal cord and becoming tetraplegic in a split second. He lost the use of his body completely from the chest down and, when he later regained some use in his fingers, that seemed to be the full extent of his recovery.

Not only was Daniel unable to walk, he was also in pain, incontinent, and suffered uncontrollable spasms in his legs and upper body. He needed twenty-four-hour care, and his mother revealed that he had tried unsuccessfully to commit suicide on three separate occasions.

Julie went straight to the heart of the dilemma she and her husband faced: 'While not everyone in Dan's situation would find it as unbearable as Dan [did], what right does any human being have to tell any other that they have to live such a life, filled with terror, discomfort and indignity?'

While Daniel's despair resonated with others who had faced sudden paralysis, there was a corresponding backlash and the Spinal Injuries Association expressed shock at Daniel's death: 'When someone has an injury like this you think it's the end of the world because life is going to change forever. But our mantra is that life need not end if you are paralysed. We know of people with similar or worse injuries than Dan who have lived fulfilling lives. A lot of people [I have] spoken to here are shocked he has taken his life.'

An inquest into Daniel James's death was opened and adjourned at the Coroner's Court in Worcestershire on 19 September. Detective Inspector Adrian Todd said, 'A police investigation is ongoing and officers have spoken with a man and a woman in connection with the case. A report will later be submitted to the Crown Prosecution Service and an inquest into the death will take place in due course.'

It would emerge that whilst the family were in Switzerland, someone had contacted the police. Faced with a similar dilemma, a concern that a family were flying to Dignitas, how many people would pick up the phone and inform the authorities? It is a decision that is far from easy and most people recognise how difficult it would be to refuse to help or support a loved one who repeatedly asks for help to end their life.

Perhaps it is fair to assume that no one can second guess what their reaction and responses will be to the sudden and irrevocable change to a family member's health. Some can learn to rebuild and reshape a life around paralysis or mobility restrictions, just as scores of those serving in the armed forces are learning to adjust after the devastating effects of roadside bombs.

Lance Corporal Tom Neathway, a sniper with the Parachute Regiment, lost both his legs and an arm after an explosion in Helmand Province in Afghanistan in 2008, the same year that Daniel took his life. Tom is from Worcester, as Daniel was, and they were a similar age when Tom was severely injured.

Tom was treated at Selly Oak and then sent for rehabilitation at Headley Court in Surrey. His progress was followed by a documentary team from the BBC. In the programme *Wounded*, Tom was under no illusion about his condition. He said, 'I was six feet tall and eleven stone. Now I'm four feet and eight stone, but I'm determined not to look like this . . . I'm not one to give up.'

It was his determination and optimism that would drive Tom Neathway's recovery. He learnt to walk on prosthetic legs in record time in order to attend his regiment's homecoming parade and collect his medal from Prince Charles. And he returned to work for the army.

Of his injuries he said, 'I was a bit gutted for about ten minutes, but there's nothing you can do, so I just focused on getting up as soon as I possibly could. I've not been devastated by it; my parents found it a hell of a lot worse than I have, but seeing how I've reacted they can't be down in the dumps whatsoever.'

Tom Neathway is a truly impressive young man and his approach to managing life with his disabilities is an inspiration to many. But not everyone who finds their life changed forever can find that same resolve as Tom and it is unfair to expect it of them.

And if they can't, what then . . . ?

The moral difficulty for many was that, despite his complete inability to move or care for himself, despite the pain, discomfort, incontinence and humiliation which he felt so deeply, Daniel James was not suffering from a terminal disease.

Dr Peter Saunders of the Care Not Killing Alliance said, 'This young man, Daniel James, did not need help to kill himself: he needed help to live with severe disability.

'It is most unfortunate that he fell into the hands of Dignitas when he did. He was still very much in the acute stage of loss and he was also almost certainly profoundly depressed. It is a terrible tragedy.'

Inevitably, this pronouncement sparked an answering

response from Dignity in Dying. Dr Michael Irwin, a retired GP and former medical director of the United Nations said, 'It had to be his choice and I would not in any way condemn this young man's parents.'

Dr Irwin, who had three times accompanied people to Dignitas, said it was clear that the British authorities were content to take no action unless there was evidence to show a death was anything other than voluntary.

Dr Irwin supports assisted suicide, but it is interesting to note that he too is unclear about what direction the law should take next. He believes that 'the law, in a sense, should stay as it is because there might be a case of someone who is tricked into going to Dignitas by their relatives and therefore, in that case, police might feel they should start an inquiry and take some action afterwards.'

The fear is that we may inadvertently move from what Baroness Campbell characterised as 'from red to green'. As Peter Saunders cautions, 'At Dignitas we started with people with cancer and motor neurone disease, then we went to chronically ill people, and those with conditions such as diabetes or multiple sclerosis where their life expectancy isn't necessarily shortened.

'Now we are moving on to people with severe disabilities. It is turning into a copycat scenario and it disturbs me. It is right for the police to investigate these cases.'

*

On 20 October it was announced that material from the investigation into Daniel's death was to be passed on to the Crown Prosecution Service's Complex Casework Unit. The CPS said the case would be reviewed by the special unit, based in Birmingham, which dealt with high-profile complex crimes, once the police had completed their inquiry.

A CPS spokesman said, 'The head of the Complex Casework Unit will review the police file and then make a decision on whether to proceed with a prosecution or not.'

In the second week of December, Keir Starmer QC, the Director of Public Prosecutions and the key figure in the entire discussion on mercy killings and assisted suicides, reported in detail on Daniel's case and its aftermath. It gave a fascinating insight into the workings of Dignitas and its processes – processes which Daniel followed that would eventually allow him to end his life. The report also reveals some of the emotional torment that his mother and father had to endure.

Daniel was diagnosed as tetraplegic, paralysed from the chest down and with no independent hand or finger movement, albeit he retained normal mobility and strength in his shoulders, biceps and triceps, the DPP said. By November 2007, the consultant had concluded that it was unlikely there would ever be any significant improvement in Daniel's neurological status, saying, 'There is no cure for complete spinal cord injury at this stage and unfortunately there is no treatment available to either aid or produce recovery.'

The DPP's detailed analysis of the case was relevant not just to Daniel's death, but to other cases as well:

'The impact of his injuries on Daniel was profound. In the early months he gave his all to prove the medical prognosis incorrect, but ultimately he came to accept that his condition would never improve.

'Daniel became suicidal, driven by his distress at his predicament and his dependency on others. To his consultant psychiatrist, he described himself as a "dynamic, active, sporty young man who loved travel and being independent" and said that he "could not envisage a worthwhile future for himself now". Daniel frequently stated his wish that he had died of his injuries on the rugby field and that he was determined to end his own life. He made several attempts to do so.

'One week after a third failed suicide attempt, Daniel contacted Dignitas in Switzerland on 20 February 2008 asking for assistance in dying. As he put it in his own words, "The primary reason I wish for your help is simply that I want to die, and due to my disability I am unable to make this happen [. . .] Not a day has gone by without [my] hoping it will be my last [. . .] I do not want another failed attempt." Dignitas sent him a welcome letter and a statement of account.

'On 9 May 2008, Dignitas wrote to Daniel to inform him that a local doctor had considered his case and had given consent for the necessary barbiturate prescription to be written. The letter explained the options available. Daniel chose to meet the local doctor twice in three days and then undergo the assisted suicide procedure on the day following the second meeting.

'On 25 July 2008, Dignitas again wrote to Daniel requesting him to sign and return an authorisation form and, on the same date, his schedule was sent to him. The final procedure would be carried out at a Dignitas apartment at eleven a.m. on Friday, 12 September.

'During the making of these arrangements, various individuals, including Daniel's parents and health professionals, tried in vain to persuade him to change his mind. Daniel remained resolute that no professional body could help him and that no-one would change his mind.

'As his psychiatrist wrote in a report dated 2 July 2008, Daniel James "clearly understood that no other parties, be they professionals or family members, wished him to pursue this course of action and was clearly aware that he could reverse his decision at any point. He remained firmly of the opinion that support from any agency would not be helpful for him or change his decision." '

The DPP then referred to the plight of Mrs James and her husband – a drama that would be enacted again in other cases.

'Daniel's parents were particularly distressed by his wish to end his own life,' the DPP said, 'and tried relentlessly to persuade him not to do so.'

As Daniel's father put it in interview, 'We pleaded with him not to do it and change his mind and live [. . .] we were all so upset but at the end of the day it was what he wanted.' Later he added, 'Even up to the last second [. . .] I hoped he'd change his mind, and my wife – I know she felt exactly the same. There would be nobody happier to hear him say he'd changed his mind and he didn't want to do it.'

However, Daniel's parents came to accept his wish to travel to Switzerland to commit suicide and, although it was against their own wishes, they began to assist him in his correspondence with Dignitas. They also agreed to accompany Daniel and to that end they organised flights and arranged for appropriate carers to be available to assist their son with his daily routine.

From a very early stage a family friend had offered assistance to Daniel. What he initially had in mind was organising flights for Daniel to see consultants anywhere in the world if that became necessary. Once Daniel had determined that he wanted to go to Switzerland to end his life, his parents took up the offer of assistance. The friend arranged a flight from Bristol to Zurich. He also booked a return flight in case Daniel changed his mind.

Daniel and his parents attended the two consultations in Switzerland as arranged, during which most of the discussion was between Daniel and the doctor. It remained clear that Daniel would not change his mind.

Daniel had been assessed by a consultant psychiatrist on a number of occasions. In her report dated 31 January 2008, the psychiatrist observed that

'Daniel's parents stated clearly that they had now come to accept his wish to die. It was evident that they were not planning to assist Daniel and would ensure that obvious means of suicide were kept out of Daniel's way, but were prepared to accept the responsibility that Daniel may at some future point attempt or succeed to take his own life at home.'

The psychiatrist saw him again on 22 February 2008. She spent an hour with Daniel, who was clear about his wish to die, and was also clear that this was not something he wanted to do by his own hand, particularly for the sake of his family, unless there was no other option available to him. In her report, dated 11 March 2008, the consultant psychiatrist concluded, 'In summary, with the benefit of having assessed Daniel on several occasions over a period of time, I am of the opinion that he has full capacity to make decisions about his medical treatment. He is fully aware of the reality and potential finality of his decision, displays clear, coherent, logical thinking processes in order to arrive at his decision and has clearly weighed alternatives in the balance.'

Following Daniel's acceptance by Dignitas, doctors carried out a review of his condition and agreed that he had the capacity to make decisions with regard to medical treatment, and that his decision to engage Dignitas was not driven by a mental illness.

On 27 August 2008 Daniel signed a declaration, witnessed by his doctor, that he wished to travel to Switzerland for an assisted suicide and for his body subsequently to be returned to England.

On 12 September 2008 he attended the clinic with his parents where a doctor helped him to take his own life. His parents were with him when he died. A death certificate confirmed that Daniel's death was 'non-natural'.

His body was not subjected to a full forensic post-mortem examination on his return to the UK, but post-mortem blood samples were analysed and disclosed a fatal level of a form of barbiturate typically used for this type of procedure in Zurich.

The DPP then addressed what steps he could, if he chose, take against Mark and Julie James and the family friend who had helped them.

He said that under Section 2(1) of the Suicide Act 1961 *a person who aids, abets, counsels or procures the suicide of another, or an attempt by another to commit suicide, shall be liable on conviction on indictment to imprisonment for a term not exceeding fourteen years.*

'In order to prove the offence of aiding and abetting Daniel's suicide,' stated Keir Starmer, 'it would be necessary to prove, firstly, that he took his own life and, secondly, that an individual or individuals had aided and abetted Daniel in committing suicide.

'The fact of the suicide can be established by the evidence and I am satisfied that these elements enable the conclusion properly to be drawn that, beyond reasonable doubt, Daniel James died as a result of suicide.

'The mental element that has to be proved is an intention to do the acts which the individual in question knew to be capable of helping, supporting or assisting suicide. The question is therefore whether by their various acts Daniel's parents or the family friend did, in fact, help, support or assist Daniel James to commit suicide and whether, when they did so, they knew that their acts were capable of helping, supporting or assisting him to do so.'

Mr Starmer then turned specifically to the role of Daniel's parents. 'Although it is necessary to examine the actions that each suspect/defendant has taken, it is clear that the actions of Daniel's parents were taken jointly. There is not absolute clarity from their interviews as to which of them did what, but there is compelling evidence of joint enterprise.

'The acts that have taken place within the jurisdiction to aid and abet Daniel's suicide are:

1 Assisting him to send documentation etc to *Dignitas*;
2 making payments to *Dignitas* from their joint bank account;

3 making the travel arrangements to take Daniel to
   Switzerland;
4 accompanying him on the flight.

'Having considered these acts, I am satisfied that the evidential test under the Code is met. Against that background, I have decided that, although neither of them assisted in the act of suicide itself, there is, on a purely objective analysis, enough evidence to provide a "realistic prospect of conviction" against Daniel's parents under Section 2(1) Suicide Act 1961.'

Then, addressing the role of the family friend, the DPP said, 'His involvement is significantly less than that of Daniel's parents. However, for the same reasons as apply to them, I have decided that his actions in arranging the flights and paying for those flights, knowing the purpose of the visit to Switzerland, are sufficient to provide a realistic prospect of conviction against him in relation to an offence of aiding and abetting Daniel James to commit suicide.'

So, should Mark and Julie be prosecuted? The DPP had made clear that there was enough evidence to proceed, but then he said, 'Neither Mark and Julie James nor the family friend influenced Daniel James to commit suicide. On the contrary, his parents tried relentlessly to persuade him not to commit suicide. Daniel was a mature, intelligent and fiercely independent young man with full capacity to make decisions about his medical treatment.

There is clear evidence that he had attempted to commit suicide on three occasions and that he would have made further attempts if and whenever an opportunity to do so arose. On the facts of this case, these are factors against prosecution.

'Although the evidential test under the Code is met, a wide range of conduct of varying degrees of culpability is caught by Section 2(1) Suicide Act 1961 and, although not truly minor acts [. . .] were towards the less culpable end of the spectrum. That is a factor against prosecution.

'Neither Daniel's parents nor the family friend stood to gain any advantage, financial or otherwise, by his death. On the contrary, for his parents, Daniel's suicide has caused them profound distress. That is a factor against prosecution.

'Taking those factors into account [. . .] I have decided that the factors against prosecution clearly outweigh those in favour. In the circumstances I have concluded that a prosecution is not needed in the public interest.'

In other words, there had been a two-stage test applied by prosecutors when deciding whether to prosecute: whether sufficient evidence existed, *and* whether it would be in the public interest to take the case to trial.

Keir Starmer's interpretation of the issues represented the first significant decision he had made since taking over as head of the Crown Prosecution Service at the end of October. In delivering his decision, he said, 'This is a tragic case, involving as it does the death of a young man in difficult and unique circumstances. While there are public interest factors in favour of prosecution, not least of which is the seriousness of this offence, I have determined that these are outweighed by the public interest factors that say that a prosecution is not needed.

'In reaching my decision I have given careful consideration to the Code for Crown Prosecutors. In particular, but not exclusively, I would point to the fact that Daniel, as a fiercely independent young man, was not influenced by his parents to take his own life and the evidence indicates he did so despite their imploring him not to.

'I send my condolences to Daniel's family and friends.'

The day after the DPP's decision was announced, an inquest was held into Daniel's death. His father described the agony that any loving parent feels at having to deal with the nightmare of having a child so critically ill.

Mark James told the inquest of the events leading up to Daniel taking a dose of lethal medication. He said the family met Dignitas staff in an apartment. 'We sat around a table and they explained to Dan what was going to happen. They asked several times if that was what he wished. They said to him, "If you take this drink you will die." They asked if he wanted to stop. Dan said, "No, I would like to carry on." The drink was brought and placed in front of him, then he took it on his own.'

Mr James explained how his son was assessed by doctors before being given the drugs to ensure he was mentally sound and capable of making his decision: 'We had to take Dan to see a doctor over there on two occasions and there had to be a break between seeing the doctor. They had to interview Dan to find out that everything was as Dan said it was.'

The Worcestershire coroner Geraint Williams said that he had asked for blood samples to be produced when Daniel's body was returned to Britain. He concluded that the cause of Daniel's death was a fatal dose of the drug pentobarbitone. Recording a verdict of suicide, the coroner said, 'A suicide must never be presumed, it must always be proven. I have to be satisfied that Daniel intended to take his life and then took an action to achieve that end.

'Daniel travelled to a clinic in Switzerland. He died on September 12th, 2008 in Zurich, Switzerland. In light of information I have heard, I have no doubt of Dan's intention and therefore record the verdict that Daniel Mark James killed himself.'

Addressing Daniel's parents, Geraint Williams added, 'There is nothing a coroner can say to make your loss any easier. Please accept my condolences.'

Outside the court, family solicitor Adrian Harling read out a statement on behalf of Daniel's parents:

'My clients would like to thank all for the support they have had throughout this heartbreaking ordeal. They are not campaigners or fighting a case for euthanasia or assisted suicide, they purely helped their son carry out his wish.

'If he had not suffered from his disabilities they would not in any event have allowed him to make that journey alone.

'My clients hopes the decision may help others in a similar situation. However, every case is different.'

9

The Last Words

—

No-one would better understand the torment that Lynn Gilderdale went through than her mother, Kay. Day after day, month after month, year after endless year, her daughter lay in that back bedroom, isolated from the rest of the world.

There was one tool, however, by which Lynn could communicate beyond the walls of that room, one way to connect with the outside world. That tool is a website called *LiveJournal*.

LiveJournal, frequently abbreviated to *LJ*, is a virtual community where internet users can keep a blog. Available in over thirty languages and with over 350,000 users in the UK alone, for Lynn in her latter years it became a source of contact with events beyond the circumscribed universe of her room.

Under the pseudonym 'Jessie Oliver', she would use her specially designed handheld computer to go onto the networking forum and share her thoughts on whatever subject she chose. Lynn's character and personality shone through in the journal: bright and thoughtful, and very supportive to those she made contact with.

Friendships developed online and, eventually, Lynn decided that she would share with these friends her toughest of all decisions: her desire to die.

Bedridden and robbed of the power of speech for all of her adolescent and adult life, she had decided by this stage that she was never going to recover, but she wanted to make sure her life would end before she lost all dignity.

The revelations about her thoughts and her decision were made to her parents and her small group of friends in the last two years of her life. Many but by no means all of those she communicated with were, like her, girls and women of all ages who also suffered from ME and had been confined to bed or housebound for years as a result.

'She did mention to me and a very few others that she had an overwhelming desire to die,' said Emily Levick. 'I recall the time I first read about it. I cried, and then immediately texted her, as she was so afraid that her friends would think badly of her for it, and I wanted to reassure her that I could never think badly of her.

'She had battled for so many years, and was so desperately tired. It was quite literally heartbreaking to read something like that, but I did understand her reasons. I believe I would have felt exactly the same if I were in her situation.'

Kay and Richard were, as we know, heartbroken by Lynn's decision to die, and her friends believe that it would have appalled her to think that her loving mother would be prosecuted and have to endure a lengthy legal battle for helping her daughter to follow her wishes.

Lynn frequently described her love for her mother in e-mails and texts to friends online. During one of her many hospital visits, she wrote on *LJ* to a friend, saying, 'You asked if my parents are able to visit and the answer is they actually never leave my side. One of them's ALWAYS here and Mum sleeps here too.'

On her thirty-first birthday in September 2008, three months before she died, Lynn told her mother how very much she would like to hear her online friends' voices, given that she couldn't physically meet them. After that conversation, and unbeknownst to Lynn, Kay e-mailed a number of Lynn's friends to arrange a surprise. When it was all done, Lynn watched videos prepared by some friends, and listened to voice messages from others. It was a profoundly meaningful experience for her.

With the passing of time, Lynn's communications online had become increasingly desperate. In 2006 she had begun talking about ending her life. 'I'm tired, so very, very tired,' she wrote on one occasion. 'I can't keep hanging on to an ever-diminishing hope that I might one day be well again [. . .] My spirit is broken,' she said, adding she would seize the opportunity to leave the world 'with both hands'.

*

After Kay's trial ended, Lynn's online diary was released, revealing the suffering she, her mother, and the rest of her loved ones, had had to endure.

Reading it gives both a glimpse and some insight into the life she and her mother shared:

OK guys, I have something really important to say. I want to talk about something extremely private and personal to share with you, my closest friends. After many years of serious deliberation, I have pretty much come to a huge decision. I hope you will try to understand my reasons for this decision and even if you don't personally agree with it I hope you won't judge me too harshly.

I don't know how to begin. I am just going to come out with it. Here goes, deep breaths. Basically I think some of you have known for a while I have had enough of this miserable excuse for a life, of merely semi-existing for the last 16 years. I have had enough and I want to die. This is no whim and certainly not just because of the reactive depression diagnosed a few months ago. I am no longer on antidepressants because they weren't doing anything for me.

I really, really, really want to die and have had enough of being so sick and in so much pain every second of every day and, basically, one serious health crisis after another. I am tired, so very, very tired and I just don't think I can keep hanging on for that elusive illness-free existence.

I can't keep hanging on for that ever diminishing nonexistent hope that one day I will be well again. This is something I have thought long and hard about, and more than once about. I'm sure it's what I want. I have discussed and continued to discuss with my parents at great length. Although they obviously desperately don't want me to go, they can see I have just had enough and understand why I can't keep hanging on for much longer.

A few months ago, some pretty extreme situations arose. Something happened here and I was finally tipped over the edge. I tried to end my life by sticking a syringe straight down into my veins and simultaneously a syringe full of air. This was not a desperate cry for help, it was a serious attempt to end my life. It should have been enough to kill a grown man. No, it didn't finish me off. Eventually, I have become tolerant to morphine after being on it for years.

All the overdose did was render me unconscious for a few hours until I finally felt Dad shaking me awake.

That was really the first time my parents knew how depressed I was. I had managed to hide it by using my time-worn, fake-happy face, when they are around. I begged my parents not to tell the doctor what I had done. But I was put on antidepressants.

Drugs have stopped me from crying all the time, but it hasn't stopped me from my desire not be on this planet any more. Nothing can change my mind. I have since promised I won't try to kill myself again in secret.

Injecting morphine is the only reliable suicide method I have access to myself. There's no other possible way to do it on my own.

Dad, he has always hated me talking about it in the past. He was quite heartbroken. He said, 'I understand. But what would I do without my best mate?' This made me sob even harder than I already had.

After talking to me for ages, they both were extremely reluctant but agreed that if something life-threatening did happen to me they promised that they would inform the doctors and nurses that I didn't want to be revived in any circumstances. I refuse to go back for more treatment.

I know there is a slim chance that I could fully recover and live a relatively normal life but even if I wake up tomorrow, I still won't be able to live the life I dreamt about living.

My ovaries have packed up — I won't be able to have children, my all time favourite wish.

I am already 31 years old. By the time I have found the man I want to have children with I will be far past the age. I cannot see myself ever being well enough to do any of this.

Also my bones are so osteoporotic that every cough and sneeze could cause a fracture. How can I live the life I have dreamed of; swimming, sailing, running, cycling. The kind of life I had before it was taken away from me at the age of 14.

My body is tired and my spirit is broken. I have had enough. Can you understand that? I hope you can, I really, really do.

In addition to not wanting any lifesaving treatment, if I am ever presented with an opportunity to leave this world, I have to admit I will grab it with both hands.

I understand people think I am just depressed or worse — suicide is far from easy in my opinion and recent experience — or they think it is ridiculous thinking of suicide when there is still a chance I could recover.

I am also painfully aware that I have a couple of special friends with their own terrible diseases.

I was 30 last year, the desire to leave all this pain and sadness behind me has nothing but increased. I want to die so, so much. Mum and I have probably spent hours on and off discussing everything, despite her doing her best to make me see things differently my resolve to leave this life has done nothing but intensify.

I am sorry. I know this may be a shock to some of you. Try to put yourself in my situation. Read all the newspaper articles online. This is only a tiny part of what I have been through in the past 16 years.

To see what every second of life in intense pain, feeling permanently and extremely ill, not just lying in a bed resting but 100 per cent reliance on others to care for my basic needs. I have survived because of tubes of medicine, pumps and drugs. Without all this modern technology I wouldn't be here.

Imagine you lived in one small room, in one single bed for 16 years since the age of 14.

Imagine being 30 years old and never having kissed someone properly. Yep, I am that pathetic 30-year-old virgin that everyone ridicules.

Imagine having the painful bones of a 100-year-old woman unable to move without risking a fracture.

Imagine being unable to get the spinning thoughts out of your head, other than by slowly typing e-mails.

Imagine not being able to turn yourself over in bed or move your legs.

Imagine having to use a bed pan lying down and having your mother wipe your bum for you.

Imagine having never been in a pub or club at 31 years old.

Imagine never having been able to fulfil one thing above all else — that thing that should be a right for all young women, the right to have a young child. I know some women are unable to, but it doesn't stop my heart from aching and the need to hold my own baby.

Imagine being imprisoned inside the miserable existence that is your life.

I don't have to imagine any of that. My body and mind are broken. I am so desperate to end the never-ending carousel of pain and sickness and suffering. I love my family. I have nothing left and I am spent.

How are Mum and Dad coping with all this? They are utterly, utterly heartbroken, naturally. Although I fear they won't get over losing me and they don't want me to go, and despite all the pain they must be in every time I discuss this whole thing, they must understand why I've had enough of this life and can't keep hanging on. They both said they would either die or feel the same. I am so lucky to have incredible parents.

I desperately want to die. Mum and Dad know I have made up my mind.

They have made sure repeatedly that this is what I truly want. And now I'm not going to resist temptation if a way of ending my life falls into my lap.

Even though I can't imagine how hard this must be for them, obviously they won't want to lose me but they can't bear for me to suffer any more than I have — that's true unconditional love. I will never be able to thank them for putting my needs above theirs. However sad it is, it's going to be my time to go very soon.

November 2008: I am afraid I can't lie. I still do crave suicide with every fibre of my being. I promised my parents that I won't attempt to do it in secret again. If the chance falls into my lap I will grab it with both hands. Mum regularly goes through everything with me. I never waver, I just become more and more sure as time passes. I have always stated that if I was unable to make a decision myself the power goes jointly to my parents. I trust them implicitly with my life and death. I know they won't do the selfish thing in keeping me here purely for themselves.

It is impossible to read Lynn Gilderdale's words without feeling how much has been lost. She was a kind and intelligent woman who should have been able to seize life with both hands, not left hunting for the solace of death as an end to suffering.

Within a short time of her death becoming public knowledge, the following message of sympathy was posted on *LiveJournal*:

> Those who met her in real life after she became ill have documented what they saw; a girl who could not speak, who could not move from her bed, her body broken by severe ME and forced into meltdown by the intervention of misguided medical professionals. Those with little or no understanding of the critical importance of total rest during the initial stages of sudden-onset, acute ME. Those of us who knew her online knew a different Lynn. We knew a bright, intelligent and optimistic girl with a lively spirit and a keen sense of humour who always had a kind word of support whenever one of us was feeling low.
>
> Yesterday I discovered I'd lost a dear friend. I know that for Lynn it was the release she had desperately craved. For me and the rest of her friends her passing has left a huge heart-shaped hole in all our lives.

10

A Good Death

⁓

The debate on how far society was willing to allow mothers such as Kay Gilderdale and Frances Inglis to end the agony of their seriously ill children was now occupying the thoughts of the highest in the land. So much so that Prime Minister Gordon Brown entered the debate.

As prosecutors were preparing to introduce guidelines to ease the plight of those who help others to end their lives so that they might be able to do so without facing criminal charges, the Prime Minister warned against legalising assisted suicide. He said such a change to the law would create the risk of putting the frail and ill under pressure to end their lives.

His warning came a day before DPP Keir Starmer was to set out the long-awaited final guidelines on assisted suicide. He was widely expected to make it clear that those who helped others end their lives were unlikely to face court action if it was clear that they acted solely out of compassion. Many saw that as effectively decriminalising assisted suicide, but the argument was far from over.

Gordon Brown had consistently opposed legislative changes on assisted suicide, and the strength and timing of his remarks were interpreted by some as a signal to Mr Starmer not to go too far. There was simmering tension too between the role of the executive – Parliament should determine any changes to the law on a matter as significant as this – and the scope of the judiciary. However, the Prime Minister said, 'It is for him [Starmer] to clarify his approach and the Government has not made any representation to him.'

Mr Starmer knew that the guidelines were necessary. Cases such as that of Debbie Purdy demanded clarity as to the circumstances in which someone was likely to be charged if they helped another person to die. The issue was obviously one that extended far beyond the role and actions of mothers such as Frances and Kay; others, such as husbands or wives, also faced end-of-life decisions. Assisted suicide had become a legal minefield, and lawyers had pointed out that there was no precedent for prosecutors to set out in such detail how people could commit a crime without being charged.

The fact that Gordon Brown was involving himself in the debate demonstrated the impact of the mounting number of cases that were being reported and discussed in the media. Writing in the *Daily Telegraph*, the Prime Minister was possibly correct in saying, 'I believe that people are drawn to support the right to assisted suicide because of fears about how they will be cared for when they are dying.

'They ask themselves, Will I be left alone? Will I suffer pain? Will I lose my dignity and my individuality? Will there be no one there to care for me? Will I be kept alive and subjected to tests and treatments that will do little good and serve only to extend the process of dying?'

No doubt it is right to assume that the question of 'a good death' is a concern not only for our loved ones but also for ourselves. Mr Brown is an admirer of Dame Cicely Saunders, the nurse who later became a physician and who pioneered the foundation of hospices for the terminally ill. Dame Cicely became committed to the advancement of pain management early in her nursing career, and in the late 1950s she began researching into how medication could best be used to relieve physical suffering.

Palliative care, as it became known, was ultimately adopted as a cornerstone of caring for the terminally and chronically ill. Her compassion and pioneering approach meant that thousands upon thousands of patients gained access to pain control medication, which allowed them and their families to ease the onset of what would have otherwise been a traumatic and painful death.

Dame Cicely was a devout Christian whose beliefs informed her professional life, but she more than understood the difficulties that come with loss. In one year, 1960, she lost her father, a close friend, and the man she loved. She later recalled the crisis she faced as one of 'pathological grieving'. Death, however, is an inescapable part of living and, like all aspects of life, it can be approached as something to be managed.

The medical advances made over the years since Dame Cicely Saunders qualified as a doctor are remarkable, but they have also meant for some – like Frances Inglis, for example – that patients are surviving the kind of serious accidents that may well have ended lives thirty or forty years earlier.

These advances in medicine have brought with them a new set of ethical dilemmas. Individuals are now faced with a loved one whose life is extended beyond their ability to communicate their wishes as to how what remains of that life should be managed. Added to the problem is a lack of confidence in standards of patient care in the health system.

The concern that staff do not have enough time to properly care for patients has even become a worry to nursing staff themselves. A survey of employees of East Lancashire NHS Trust in 2010 revealed that fifty-two percent would not want their own family members or friends to be in their care, in the hospitals they work in. Whilst care standards are often high and the attitude of nursing staff praised, it is not unheard of for people to find that their relatives have been left lying neglected in a ward, thirsty, hungry and even lying in their own excretions.

Yet knowing that a loved one 'would not have wanted'

to be kept alive and in a condition that requires round-the-clock care is simply not sufficient ground to end another person's life. It would be all too easy for such an understanding to be open to abuse.

In September 2009, the Director of Public Prosecutions published an interim policy on prosecuting assisted suicides. Keir Starmer clarified what the new guidelines would mean and his remarks revealed a key shift in focus. 'The policy,' he said, 'is now more focused on the motivation of the suspect rather than the characteristics of the victim.

'The policy does not change the law on assisted suicide. It does not open the door for euthanasia. It does not override the will of Parliament. What it does is to provide a clear framework for prosecutors to decide which cases should proceed to court and which should not.

'Assessing whether a case should go to court is not simply a question of adding up the public interest factors for and against prosecution and seeing which has the greater number. It is not a tick-box exercise. Each case has to be considered on its own facts and merits.

'As a result of the consultation exercise there have been changes to the policy. But that does not mean prosecutions are more or less likely. The policy has not been relaxed or tightened but there has been a change of focus.'

Starmer had to allay fears that vulnerable people would be pressured into taking their own lives. From a practical point of view, the policy set out the key factors likely to lead to those who assist in suicide facing court action. They outline a sensible assessment of why a prosecution *would* be favoured and they are worth noting:

- The victim was under 18 years of age;
- the victim's capacity to reach an informed decision was adversely affected by a recognised mental illness or learning difficulty;
- the victim did not have a clear, settled and informed wish to commit suicide; for example, the victim's history suggests that his or her wish to commit suicide was temporary or subject to change;
- the victim did not indicate unequivocally to the suspect that he or she wished to commit suicide;
- the victim did not ask personally on his or her own initiative for the assistance of the suspect;
- the victim did not have a terminal illness; or a severe and incurable physical disability; or a severe degenerative physical condition from which there was no possibility of recovery;
- the suspect was not wholly motivated by compassion; for example, the suspect was motivated by the prospect that they or a person closely connected to them stood to gain in some way from the death of the victim;
- the suspect persuaded, pressured or maliciously encouraged the victim to commit suicide, or exercised

improper influence in the victim's decision to do so;
and did not take reasonable steps to ensure that any
other person did not do so.

Reaction to the guidelines came from a variety of organisations. Jayne Spink, director of policy and research at the MS (Multiple Sclerosis) Society, said, 'While we welcome the guidance and the clarity it provides, we remain concerned that the law on assisted suicide continues to place a burden on individuals to seek end of life care and support themselves, rather than on society to provide it.'

Richard Hawkes, chief executive of disability charity Scope, warned, 'We do not support any weakening of the protection offered under the law on assisted suicide, which is exactly what these new guidelines do. Many disabled people are frightened by the consequences of these new guidelines and with good reason. There is a real danger these changes will result in disabled people being pressured to end their lives.'

Groups in favour of assisted dying suggested the guidance did not go far enough because what was needed was a clear change in the law. Sarah Wootton, chief executive of Dignity in Dying, welcomed the guidelines as a 'victory for common sense and compassion' but added that the charity remained committed to pressing for a change in the law.

Members of Parliament demanded a full debate so that Parliament, rather than the DPP, would shape policy.

Labour MP David Winnick emphasised the importance of debating the policy 'in view of the controversy', and Conservative MP Mark Pritchard believed it was up to Parliament to set the law and to the courts to interpret it: 'There is real concern out in the community,' he said, 'that this House is not having a say. People are very concerned that this is a new back door to euthanasia in the UK.'

Debbie Purdy who had campaigned to try and protect her husband from prosecution, naturally had a vested interest in the new focus of the guidelines. She felt that 'The important thing about the guidelines is they've been able to really clarify the difference between malicious encouragement and compassionate support for somebody's decision.' She added, 'Keir Starmer and the CPS have done the best they can in bringing the 1961 Suicide Act [up to date, and] how it will be interpreted in the twenty-first century. It's fifty years old, we live in a different world.'

In this different world, the United Kingdom is not the only country struggling to find an acceptable balance between the rights of an individual and protection of the vulnerable. In the United States, each state can take a view on how best to protect their citizens, and the state of Oregon has become a beacon for those looking for a more 'enlightened' approach.

In Oregon, after consultation with two doctors, the terminally ill patient is given a prescription that will end their life. What is interesting is that four out of ten of those who have the prescription die without having used it. The issue for so many is one of control; knowing that the prescription is to hand allows them the comfort of choice – a point forcibly made by Debbie Purdy.

Overall, organisations on both sides of the debate welcomed the guidelines. Lord Carlile QC, chairman of Care Not Killing, said that they 'greatly reduce the risk of undermining existing law.' But Dr Peter Saunders of the same campaign group, while acknowledging that the final rules were an improvement on those previously published in September, added this chilling note: 'How will a prosecutor decide if someone's motives are wholly compassionate? How can he tell? The key witness is dead.'

Can you trust the testimony of someone who could possibly avoid prosecution by lying about what they did?

The true test of these guidelines will be their application in practice as new cases arise. For the present, assisting or encouraging suicide is still a crime and carries a sentence of up to fourteen years. This can only be changed by an Act of Parliament.

And despite all efforts to clarify the law as it stands, those who find themselves wishing to assist a loved one to commit suicide may still feel that going to Dignitas in Switzerland offers the best protection. More than a hundred Britons have ended their lives in the Dignitas clinics, and not one of their relatives has been successfully prosecuted.

The guidelines have since seen some changes. For example, the DPP dropped some of the most controversial provisions, such as that prosecutors were not to pursue those who helped the disabled or dying to kill themselves. Campaigners had protested against those clauses and Mr Starmer, accepting the argument that they could discriminate against the disabled, removed them.

Proposals for more lenient treatment for close relatives also went, following protests that spouses and family members can act out of malice or greed.

Mr Starmer emphasised that mercy killing remained classified as murder, and that all cases where someone is suspected of assisting a suicide would be fully investigated. Medical personnel, pro-suicide campaigners, clinic owners, those who help children and youngsters to die, violent bullies, and those who try to persuade someone to kill themselves would all face trial.

The DPP also pointed out that, 'The offence of encouraging or assisting suicide carries a maximum penalty of 14 years' imprisonment. This reflects the seriousness of the offence. Committing or attempting to commit suicide is not, however, of itself, a criminal offence [. . .]

'The case of *Purdy* did not change the law: only Parliament can change the law on encouraging or assisting suicide. This policy does not in any way "decriminalise" the offence of encouraging or assisting suicide. Nothing in this policy can be taken to amount to an assurance that a person will be immune from prosecution if he or she does an act that encourages or assists the suicide or the attempted suicide of another person.'

The six public interest factors against prosecution that the DPP recommended were:

1 The victim had reached a voluntary, clear, settled and informed decision to commit suicide.
2 The suspect was wholly motivated by compassion.
3 The actions of the suspect, although sufficient to come within the definition of the crime, were of only minor encouragement or assistance.
4 The suspect had sought to dissuade the victim from taking the course of action which resulted in his or her suicide.
5 The actions of the suspect may be characterised as reluctant encouragement or assistance in the face of a determined wish on the part of the victim to commit suicide.
6 The suspect reported the victim's suicide to the police and fully assisted them in their enquiries into the circumstances of the suicide or the attempt and his or her part in providing encouragement or assistance.

As we have seen, the cases of Kay Gilderdale and Frances Inglis, although similarly tragic, differed to a great extent because Frances's actions were described as a mercy killing rather than as a case of assisting the suicide of someone who had expressed a desire to die. Her son Thomas had never had the opportunity to verbally express a wish to live or the wish to die.

Nevertheless, both the mothers' plights had touched the hearts of the nation and the reverberations, both legal and moral, continued to be felt. The facts and statements can be read, each case assessed and opinions arrived at but, in truth, should tragedy strike, families will find themselves alone with terrible decisions to make.

There is no option for a quiet, arranged and dignified death if it is to be assisted for those ill at home in the UK. As it stands, a clinic in Switzerland is still the only route open to those who wish to say enough, they will suffer no more.

11

A Fashionable Concern

It would be hard to find someone whose public image was further away from the lives led by Kay Gilderdale and Frances Inglis than best-selling author Terry Pratchett.

In December 2007 Lynn Gilderdale was, as she had been for years, lying in her quiet room in a bungalow in the middle of the English countryside; a hundred miles away Tom Inglis was in hospital after his life-threatening injury.

There had only been a handful of newspaper articles about Lynn at that time, and Frances Inglis, charged with her first attempt on her son's life, was out on bail and not yet in the public spotlight.

The same could not be said of Terry Pratchett. The son of a garage mechanic and a secretary from Beaconsfield, Buckinghamshire, he had initially been inspired to write after reading *The Wind in the Willows* and discovering that Mr Toad could drive a car. He fell in love with the book and, aged thirteen, published his first short story, 'The Hades Business', in a school magazine.

Despite the headmaster condemning the 'moral tone' of

the story, it was snapped up by a sci-fi magazine who paid £14 for it, and the youngster bought himself a second-hand typewriter with the proceeds.

Pratchett left school at sixteen to work as a reporter in local newspapers 'because it was indoor work with no heavy lifting' and later became a press officer for the Central Electricity Generation Board, dealing mainly with a nuclear power industry beleaguered by the Chernobyl disaster. He left the job when he realised that his writing was set to earn him far more than his salary at the electricity board.

He has gone on to become one of the most high-profile authors in Britain, with sales of around sixty-five million and an avid following of readers all over the world. In a BBC poll of the most loved British writers only one other author also had five books in the top one hundred: Charles Dickens. Terry Pratchett, who can also lay claim to the dubious honour of knowing that he is the 'most shoplifted author' in Britain, was awarded a knighthood in the 2009 Honours List for his services to literature.

His success lies in the fact that he is one of the few novelists to write across the adult/child divide, so much so that his work has been translated into thirty-seven languages. Sir Terry was Britain's best-selling author of the 1990s and would only be surpassed by the introduction of JK Rowling's *Harry Potter* series. His *Discworld* fantasy tales, as well as selling in vast numbers, also generate conventions and merchandising, and attract admirers bordering, in some cases, on the obsessive.

Everything that interests Pratchett – time travel, corrupt politicians, science, alchemy, collapsing postal services, dragons, goat's milk cheese, to name a few – seems to find its way into *Discworld*, his flat planet balanced on four elephants standing on a giant turtle hurtling through space. With a cast of wizards, witches, dwarfs, trolls and humans, the novels combine philosophy, humour and adventure, and have been compared to Douglas Adams's *The Hitchhiker's Guide To The Galaxy* – although some have said that Pratchett's world is closer in the scale of its vision to JRR Tolkien's Middle Earth.

In 1989, *Truckers* became the first children's book to appear in British adult fiction bestseller lists, and *The Amazing Maurice and His Educated Rodents* won the Carnegie Medal for children's fiction in 2001. He was given an OBE in 1998 for services to British literature, although he was to point out that he 'had six best-sellers before anyone thought I was worth interviewing. The feeling is that I should be pigeonholed into the category of good books for people who can't read.'

This successful and flamboyant figure, however, came to be cast in an unexpected and unwelcome role as an influential commentator in the dialogue over assisted dying, but what had he in common with the tormented mothers, and how were their lives to cross?

The first clue was spotted in the autumn of 2007 when Pratchett let slip that he had had a stroke at some stage in the previous two years, but that he hadn't been aware of it. 'I have dated it to two or three years ago, because that was when my typing started going all over the place,' he said.

He had been treated for high blood pressure and a heart condition in the past, both high-risk factors for strokes, but thought that his problems were under control and no longer a threat to his health. He had never smoked and there was no history of heart problems in his family.

But then he noticed, while working on the manuscript of a new book, 'that I was having a bad day and my typing was going askew. It was as if I was typing wearing gloves.'

He went to see his doctor. 'After going through the symptoms, the first thing she asked was whether I'd suffered any memory loss and I wisecracked back, "Not that I can recall."'

The GP gave him a basic test to rule out dementia/Alzheimer's and then referred him to a specialist, who ordered an ultrasound scan. This would show any blockages in his carotid artery, the principal artery which supplies the brain with oxygenated blood, and he also had an MRI scan to check his brain activity and see whether there were any areas of dead tissue.

Pratchett was then shown the scan. 'There were grey spots where brain cells had turned up their toes and died,' he said. The right side of the brain controls hand-eye coordination, so it seemed likely the stroke affected that side of his brain. His ability to write, controlled by the left side of the brain, was unaffected.

It seemed that he had suffered a transient ischaemic attack (TIA), a mini-stroke which can last anywhere from a few minutes to a few hours, and from which the sufferer recovers within twenty-four hours. Nonetheless, side-effects can result from brain cells being killed off. Many people are unaware that they have suffered a TIA and Sir Terry remarked, 'My speech is no less clear than before. I still have the lisp I was born with.'

He was put on cholesterol-lowering statins, gave up eating cheese, and cut down on red meat – advice on nutrition that many of us will have been urged to follow. His typing began to improve and his consultant had some reassuring news: it has been shown that it is possible for other parts of the brain to take over the functions lost to dead brain tissue.

Whilst the prognosis was by no measure bleak, soon afterwards Sir Terry noticed that he had 'forgotten' how to knot his tie. It seemed such a strange thing to have absented itself after a lifetime of automatically and unthinkingly allowing the hands, with their 'muscle memory', to execute the task. Now, standing in front of a mirror, he was mystified as to how to even begin assembling the knot.

Other developments, familiar to many of us, were less alarming. Sir Terry noted that he had become prone to saying, 'What's the name of the actress that appeared in that programme, you know the one . . . ? And later on, I shout out the name.' Being unable to retrieve a name or a date, particularly among those with a busy life, is not uncommon.

In December, however, came worrying news. Sir Terry announced on a website that he had Alzheimer's disease and, publicly at least, reacted to it in his characteristic manner and asked that those who knew and cared for him simply 'keep things cheerful'.

Alzheimer's is the most common cause of dementia, a word used to describe the symptoms that occur when the brain is affected by specific diseases and conditions. Dementia will be familiar to many since it affects over seven hundred and fifty thousand people in the UK alone and, in fifteen years' time, that number is expected to reach one million.

Alzheimer's, first described by the German neurologist Alois Alzheimer, is a physical disease affecting the brain. During its course, 'plaques' and 'tangles' develop in the structure of the brain, leading to the death of brain cells. People with Alzheimer's also have a shortage of certain important chemicals in their brains, chemicals which are involved with the transmission of messages within the brain.

It is a progressive disease, which means that gradually, over time, more parts of the brain are damaged and thus the symptoms become more severe.

Sufferers, such as Sir Terry, still in the early stages of the disease might experience lapses of memory and have problems finding the right words. Then, as the disease progresses, they can become confused and frequently forget the names of people, places, appointments and recent events. Or they can experience mood swings, perhaps feeling sad or angry as well as frightened and frustrated by their increasing memory loss. They could also become more withdrawn, due either to a loss of confidence or to communication problems.

It was another writer, the distinguished academic and novelist Iris Murdoch, who first brought the attention of the illness to the attention of the literary world. A distinguished philosopher as well as writer of fiction, she had been suffering from 'writer's block' in 1995, but subsequently learnt that her work was being impeded by the onset of Alzheimer's. She died four years later, unable to recall her many achievements.

As the illness grows worse, people with Alzheimer's need increased support from those who care for them until, eventually, they need help with all their daily activities.

There are now some drug treatments available that can at least ameliorate the symptoms or slow down the disease in some people. These drugs are not a cure, but they may stabilise some of the symptoms for a limited period of time. But there is currently no cure for dementia.

Despite the implications of the diagnosis, when Sir

Terry Pratchett publicly announced his illness on the website, he described the diagnosis as an 'embuggerance'. He added, 'Frankly, I would prefer it if people kept things cheerful, because I think there's time for at least a few more books yet.'

In the early spring of 2009 he announced a one million dollar donation to help find a cure for Alzheimer's and condemned the 'shameful' lack of funding to help fight it. He told an annual conference on Alzheimer's that having the disease was like 'stripping away your living self a bit at a time'.

At the time he spoke, the illness affected an estimated seven hundred thousand people in the UK yet only £11 per person was spent annually on research; by comparison, £289 was spent for each cancer patient.

Sir Terry's insights into his condition in some way mirror the honest and moving accounts Lynn Gilderdale gave in her journal:

'It's a nasty disease, surrounded by shadows and small, largely unseen tragedies. People don't know what to say, unless they have had it in the family. People ask me why I announced that I had Alzheimer's. My response was why shouldn't I?

'I remember when people died of "a long illness"; now we call cancer by its name and, as every wizard knows, once you have a thing's real name you have the first step to its taming.

'We are at war with cancer, and we use that vocabulary. We battle, we are brave, we survive. And we have a large armaments industry . . .

'But, on the whole, you try to be your own doctor. The internet twangs night and day. I walk a lot and take more supplements than the Sunday papers. We talk to one another and compare regimes.'

Rebecca Wood, the chief executive of the Alzheimer's Research Trust, said: 'There was an idea that it was just what happened in old age, that it was not a disease which, with enough research, could possibly be cured. What Terry is doing is challenging that mindset that there is no cure.

'He is extremely well known and very articulate so there is that celebrity element, but he, as he says, is speaking for seven hundred thousand other people with this disease who would not normally get a voice.'

Sir Terry then decided to take a stand on the controversy that would embroil him in the Gilderdale-Inglis debate: 'My view is that when there is clearly no "me" left, whatever else might be left, then painlessly disposing of the remnants would be a sensible idea.'

Prophetically, in his book *Hogfather*, adapted for television in 2006, he said of the character Death, 'Death doesn't kill people. People kill people. Old age kills people. Disease kills people. Death turns up afterwards. Indeed you can say that he is a great friend to those who are in pain. And one automatically thinks of him as caring about his job.'

In 2009 Sir Terry, as he now was, had comments to make in the wake of the House of Lords ruling that the Director of Public Prosecutions must give guidance in the Debbie Purdy application for a ruling on her husband's legal position if he were to accompany her to Dignitas.

He said, 'I live in hope I can jump before I am pushed. I believe that if the burden gets too great, those who wish should be allowed to be shown the door. In my case, in the fullness of time, I hope it will be in the garden under an English sky. Or, if wet, the library.'

Sir Terry once again emphasised that the needs of each individual do not always tarry or arrive at a comfortable accommodation. He said he had no doubt that there were people with a 'passion for caring' but asked them to accept there are people who have 'a burning passion not to need to be cared for'.

It is accepted that no one of sound mind sets out to be cruel, but as a society we are yet to establish whether we have a policy of life at any cost.

And while it is not difficult to imagine a system that accommodates the wishes of those who choose not to live with suffering and degradation, the sticking point remains how best to honour those who are unable to express their wants and needs.

*

In January 2010 it was announced that Sir Terry would become the first novelist to deliver BBC1's annual Richard Dimbleby Lecture. His speech, timely and appropriate, would tackle society's relationship with death.

Titled *Shaking Hands With Death*, Sir Terry's lecture was billed as an exploration of how modern society – confronted with an increasingly older population, many of whom will suffer from incurable illnesses – needs to redefine how it deals with death.

The Dimbleby Lecture has been given every year since 1972 by an influential public figure invited from the worlds of business or politics, or other high-profile dignitaries such as HRH the Duke of Edinburgh, Prince Charles, the Archbishop of Canterbury Dr Rowan Williams, and former US President Bill Clinton.

That Sir Terry was to be given such a platform while the controversy over the Gilderdale and Inglis trials was raging (though the timing, almost simultaneous with the verdicts was coincidental), demonstrated just how central to the public debate assisted suicide, or 'assisted death' as Sir Terry preferred it to be known, had become. And, extraordinarily, the lecture, broadcast live on BBC1, was delivered on the same night and the same TV channel that the *Panorama* programme about Kay and Lynn Gilderdale, complete with its public opinion poll, was transmitted.

The Dimbleby Lecture was held in the library of the Royal College of Physicians. Sir Terry spoke only briefly before the actor Tony Robinson, his 'stunt Pratchett', read his words – an impassioned plea that assisted death 'is an idea whose time is really coming' and calling for a tribunal to be set up where people can apply for legal permission to end their lives at a time of their choosing.

Although the starting point was personal – Alzheimer's and its impact on him – Sir Terry's entire speech was relevant to the deaths of Lynn Gilderdale and Tom Inglis, two young people who should have been in the prime of life but who, for differing reasons, had been dealt terrible blows by fate.

When he spoke of the death of his own father, who suffered a protracted end due to pancreatic cancer, Sir Terry reflected the fears of many: 'On the day he was diagnosed my father told me, "If you ever see me in a hospital bed, full of tubes and pipes and no good to anybody, tell them to switch me off."

'In fact, it took something under a fortnight in the hospice for him to die as a kind of collateral damage in the war between his cancer and the morphine. And in that time he stopped being him and started becoming a corpse, albeit one that moved ever so slightly from time to time . . .

'He did not want to die a curious kind of living death. He wasn't that kind of person. He wanted to say goodbye to me, and knowing him, he would probably have finished with a joke of some sort. And if the nurses had put the relevant syringe in the cannula, I would have pressed it, and felt it was my duty. There would have been tears, of course there would; tears would be appropriate and insuppressible.'

Sir Terry Pratchett's observations and sentiments were all too human. Each of us will have to wrestle with our own death and those of our loved ones, and each of us fears that modern medicine can mean less that we are prolonging life than extending the often painful process of dying. There is no universal approach to eliminating the hardships of what is yet to be faced, and as our expectations of our 'rights' as individuals come increasingly to the fore of the arguments, traditional morality – once the domain of the Church – seems to have been pushed to the sidelines.

Perhaps then it was only right that church representatives should give their views on this burning issue.

Ancient Greece and Rome viewed self-murder as a practical step to avoid prolonged suffering but with the ascendancy of Christianity came a growing opposition to euthanasia. The Church came to argue that any life, no matter how miserable or restricted, was in possession of an immortal soul and therefore was to be cherished as having worth equal to that of any other.

The thirteenth-century Catholic theologian Thomas Aquinas summarised in three clear arguments Christianity's understanding of why suicide is wrong. First, it is contrary to nature as all living organisms strive for preservation; second it is contrary to our social obligations as 'self-murder' harms loved ones and the whole community; third God alone can decide when to end a life.

He wrote, 'To bring death upon oneself in order to escape the other afflictions of this life is to adopt a greater evil in order to avoid a lesser . . . Suicide is the most fatal of sins because it cannot be repented of.'

This was the belief that held sway for centuries. In the twenty-first century, however, the Church often finds itself at odds with the sensibilities of modern societies; whether it be the right of the State to take life as with the death penalty where it is still imposed, or the right of women to terminate an unwanted pregnancy.

Arguments about the ethics of euthanasia have not only brushed up against the rights of the terminally ill, those with degenerative illnesses and those in a persistent vegetative state, but also the question surrounding whether to keep alive very premature babies born with severe complications. Modern medicine may be able to sustain the life of babies born after less than twenty-five weeks' gestation and weighing less than two pounds, but there are now some that are voicing disquiet about what underpins the decision to do so.

It is an emotionally fraught area, as any mother who has gone into labour early will understand. Feelings of intense love and a wish to protect a child are not diminished by its early arrival. If anything, the need to ensure that all is done to help the child survive are strengthened, but research shows that very premature babies are exposed to a far higher risk of complications and it has led some doctors to speak out.

The president of the Royal College of Paediatrics, Professor Sir Alan Craft, said that many paediatricians would be in favour of not intervening to extend the lives of very young babies, that is those born at under twenty-five weeks. 'The vast majority of children born at this gestation who do survive have significant disabilities,' he added.

It is true that babies born before twenty-eight weeks have been shown to have greater health complications when compared to full-term babies, and many do face learning and developmental difficulties. For example, doctors believe that, should they survive, these babies will have a one in four chance of autism and there is an almost fifty per cent risk of cerebral palsy. In addition, a host of complications can arise associated with bowel, lung and kidney function.

It has been estimated that to raise and care for the very premature children born each year until the age of eighteen, the additional cost to the health system would be one billion pounds. Professor Sir Alan Craft raised the uncomfortable issue of financial consequences of intervention, saying, 'There is a lifetime cost and that needs to be taken into the equation when society tries to decide whether it wants to intervene.'

Needless to say, such views have been attacked by the premature babies charity Bliss who said that such views are a 'gross abuse of human rights'. Not only does this devalue the lives of those children who live with disabilities, but it also discounts the many examples of children born prematurely who have thrived.

Denying premature babies medical care is ethically repellent to the majority, but when commentators who are known for their natural compassion for others voice doubts about intervention, it does cause many to look at this difficult issue afresh.

Virginia Ironside is an 'agony aunt' with many years of experience in counselling readers faced with hardship and heartbreak. She chose to speak out on the controversial subject of premature babies in April 2010: 'Allowing these babies to die isn't an easy option – far from it. It can cause parents and families pain and guilt for years. But I believe that it can sometimes be an unselfish and loving act not to prolong the life of a child who will never leave hospital or be free from intrusive and distressing medical intervention, before he or she can suffer.'

This brings us back into the difficult territory of the decisions parents believe they can make on behalf of their children, very much as Frances Inglis did as she sat at her son's bedside.

Are a parent's instincts always correct? Strong feelings, springing from a common root of love and concern for a child, can exist at opposite ends of the spectrum. Some parents will fight for the right of a suffering child to die peacefully; others will strive for the right of their child to continue to receive medical intervention, even when doctors do not support the decision.

In March 2009, the parents of a nine-month-old baby known only at Baby OT lost their battle to keep the ventilator machine that was keeping him alive switched on. The baby had been born with a rare metabolic disorder, was brain damaged, and was unable to breathe or swallow unaided.

His doctors argued that his life was intolerable but his parents disagreed. At the High Court, one of the team treating Baby OT said, 'What we are looking at is the quality of his life. Yes, I can understand that the parents may get tremendous pleasure from their interaction with him [but] how much pain and suffering should he be made to bear when the pleasures he gets from life are few and far between?'

It would be an easier world if the medical prognoses that doctors arrive at were always infallible, but of course that isn't the case. Only three years before the Baby OT case, parents Debbie and Darren Wyatt won the right to keep their daughter Charlotte alive through the use of medical intervention. She was also brain damaged and her doctors, who gave her only a five per cent chance of survival, advised that further intervention would be detrimental. Five years later, Charlotte is still alive and is said to be learning to walk.

The Church has long preached that each life is sacred, a clear and uncompromising view that has set it on an often fraught and difficult path. When it came to speaking out on the topic of euthanasia and assisted suicide, it was the Archbishop of York, Dr John Sentamu, who criticised what some saw as a 'bandwagon of fashionable opinion' that suggested that relatives be allowed to help the sick and dying commit suicide without fear of prosecution.

Referring to the *Panorama* and *Daily Telegraph* polls, which indicated a mood in favour of change, Dr Sentamu asserted that, 'The silent majority never get asked. One thousand people out of about sixty-one million really is not very much guidance.

'Once you begin to open this particular door, it won't be long before you start having mercy killings. I would rather listen to the voices of disabled people than to the voices of celebrities or the voices of a thousand people in an opinion poll.'

He said that Parliament had twice rejected laws to legalise assisted dying, yet a euthanasia law appeared to be on the way thanks to a campaign characterised by celebrity endorsements and opinion polls.

The Church's stand on the sanctity of life, its attitude to the ideas and morality of the present arguments is entrenched in its history. However, the clear-headed approach to the issue of Sir Terry Pratchett, who has expressed the opinion and feelings of many, cannot be so easily dismissed as one of celebrity or fashion.

'I think,' Sir Terry has said, 'we should consider looking to the medical profession to do [it] with care and attention, and with understanding and with full explanation of the circumstances, to allow us to die at a time of our choosing. I think of this almost as a right. I hate the thought of amateurs helping amateurs to commit suicide.'

Sir Terry is far from the first writer or thinker to consider both the ethics and the practicalities surrounding assisted suicide. By the seventeenth and early eighteenth centuries, writers were moving away from the idea that morality required a religious foundation. In Britain, the Utilitarian thinker Jeremy Bentham argued that 'the purpose of morality is not the service of God or obedience to abstract moral rules, but the promotion of the greatest possible happiness for creatures on earth.'

These ideas were further expanded by the nineteenth-century writer, thinker and Utilitarian philosopher John Stuart Mill, who arrived at a position that will resonate with many readers today. He said that 'the individual is sovereign over his own body and mind; where one's own interests are concerned, there is no other authority.'

At face value, having sovereignty over one's own body and accepting no other authority appears a fundamental right. But the diversity of human experiences and the complexities of the human heart can cause even fixed and certain ideas to come unstuck.

Alison Davies from Dorset has struggled for many years with spina bifida. Now in her fifties, she says, 'I use a wheelchair full time and suffer severe spinal pain daily. This pain is not always well controlled, even with morphine. At its worst I can't think or speak.

'About twenty years ago, I decided I could no longer face life. I wanted to die – a strong wish that lasted for more than ten years. I attempted suicide several times.

'It took my friends years to persuade me that my life did have value. Their efforts and a trip to India in 1995, when I met disabled children, turned my life around. After that trip I remember saying I think I want to live.

'Had euthanasia been legal I would have missed the best years of my life. My life has been full of pain and suffering, true. But it has also been one long adventure. My death will also be an adventure, but for now I'll wait for it to come in its own time.'

Cases such as Alison's make us question if our assertions that we know our own minds are to be wholly trusted. Each of us has the capacity to change and renew our commitment to life even if it is now on limited physical terms. The life of the mind can still flourish.

In the wake of Sir Terry's Dimbleby Lecture and the *Panorama* programme about the Kay Gilderdale case, once more renewed resistance to a threat of a 'liberalisation' of the law was given voice. Passions run high on this topic, and a cross-party group of MPs accused the BBC of promoting euthanasia. They called on government ministers to threaten to cut off the supply of public money to the broadcaster.

An early day motion, raised by Conservative MP Ann Winterton, put before the House of Commons said the Corporation 'misused public funds' in its coverage of the issue, singling out the high profile given to Sir Terry Pratchett's lecture.

The motion claimed that the BBC 'ignored the rights of the disabled' and had used drama as well as news to promote its pro-euthanasia stance. Ann Winterton had the support of one Tory and four Labour MPs, who claimed there had been numerous complaints over the 'persistent bias of the BBC on matters relating to euthanasia and other life issues and on the manner in which the BBC has misused public funds to promote changes in the law.' The MPs complained of 'thinly disguised plays and soap operas being used to promote the use of euthanasia, and misrepresentation of pro-life activists in the UK as people of violence.' They claimed the 'multi-million pound campaign' culminated with the *Panorama* programme, and the televised Dimbleby Lecture, and said, 'As usual the BBC has ignored the rights of the disabled, despite the fact that every disability group in the UK is opposed to the legalisation of assisted suicide and euthanasia.'

They urged the Government to make it clear to the BBC that public funds would be withdrawn unless the Corporation complied with its charter and ensured that 'all programmes on issues of public interest are treated impartially.'

In response, the BBC said it was a coincidence that the *Panorama* programme was transmitted on the same evening as the Dimbleby Lecture. A spokesman said, 'The BBC takes its responsibilities very seriously, which is why we have reported these issues in a careful, balanced, and impartial way.

'We understand people hold very strong views in this area, but equally it is a legitimate topic for journalism and current affairs – it is important to report on difficult issues and not shy away from them.

'*Panorama* included an opinion poll showing that the public was evenly split on the issue of assisted suicide in cases like that of Lynn Gilderdale, and featured the views of Baroness Campbell who is against any move towards legalisation.

'The Richard Dimbleby Lecture is an annual event that has covered a range of topics over time. It is perfectly legitimate for the BBC and other news outlets to report the content of the speech, and the wide range of reactions to it.'

But the criticisms and the concern that the BBC was trying covertly to shift public perceptions and shape opinion in favour of assisted suicide did not end there.

A Liberal Democrat peer demanded a meeting with BBC chiefs over their handling of the assisted dying issue. Lord Carlile – a lawyer who acts as the independent reviewer of Government anti-terrorist law – was the most senior establishment figure to call into doubt the Corporation's reporting of assisted suicide and euthanasia.

Following complaints from MPs over coverage that some felt amounted to a campaign in favour of allowing people to kill desperately sick relatives, he asked for talks with Sir Michael Lyons, chairman of the BBC Trust, and the Corporation's Director General, Mark Thompson.

That the BBC chose to reflect on a matter of such concern to the general public is to be expected, even if the criticism it attracted was less predictable. Concerns that 'the establishment', a 'liberal elite' or, alternatively, 'celebrities' are forcing opinion to move closer to accepting a relaxation in the law is not new but is indicative of the strong feelings the topic arouses.

Despite 'fashionable' celebrity endorsement, the right to die is neither a new, nor even a recent concern, but one that actually pre-dates Christianity. Over two thousand years ago, ancient Greek philosophers engaged with the idea of suicide as a practical response to the end of one's 'care for life'.

The stoic thinker Epictetus summed up the attitude with a simple metaphor: 'If the room is smoky, if only moderately, I will stay; if there is too much smoke I will go.

Remember this, keep a firm hold on it, the door is always open.'

The reasoning seems sound and yet resistance, much of it driven by religious beliefs, meant that it was not until 1961 that the act of suicide or attempted suicide was decriminalised. Prior to that, and not surprisingly, the fact that suicide was a criminal offence never deterred those desperate enough to end their lives. But until 1961, if someone made an attempt and failed, they could be prosecuted – and so could their families.

With a change in society's understanding of 'self-murder' came a change in the law, and the fear for many campaigners in the anti camp is that the ground is set to shift once more.

The possibility that isolated victims could be coerced or browbeaten into ending their lives has remained a constant fear. A more recent area of concern adding to the argument is the worry that health and social services will buckle under the cost of providing palliative care to an increasingly elderly population. This, too, has caused some to speculate that less scrupulous relatives will persuade doctors to end prematurely the life of an elderly or infirm person. It is understandable that this alarming possibility has been raised, but it is perhaps disingenuous to imagine that health or social services professionals could be bullied so readily by grasping relatives.

However, clearly, all aspects of the issue do need to be

aired and addressed. Yet perhaps the arguments against a change in the law as it stands have overlooked one pertinent factor: even with the full weight of the law unequivocally opposed to both mercy killing and assisted suicide, neither Kay Gilderdale nor Frances Inglis was deterred from taking action.

Kay packed up her house and prepared for the worst. Frances understood that her actions fell outside the remit of the law as it stood but calmly made arrangements for the paying of bills and the feeding of her dog, and accepted that she would face arrest and prosecution.

When the heart of a mother believes, and decides, that she must put the needs of her child first, nothing will stand in her way.

12

A Question of Dignity

~

The name of one organisation in particular persistently crops up in any discussion surrounding the issue of assisting the death of a seriously or terminally ill loved one. That organisation is Dignitas.

Of the many cases that have grabbed the headlines, one of the first was that of seventy-four-year-old Reg Crew from Liverpool, a victim of motor neurone disease. He travelled to Dignitas with his wife in 2003 and became the first Briton to attract publicity for choosing to end his life at the clinic.

By the time that Kay Gilderdale and Frances Inglis stood in the dock facing criminal charges over the deaths of their children, one hundred and thirty-five Britons, including twenty-seven in 2009 alone, had flown to the affluent German-speaking city of Zurich in northern Switzerland to die at the Dignitas centre.

The British are not alone in choosing to end their lives with Dignitas. Fifty-nine per cent of those who opt for this course of action come from nearby Germany; the second largest group – fourteen per cent – are British. Irrespective of nationality, what the relatives of Dignitas clients all share is the agonising dilemma over the timing and means of their loved one's death.

As well as concerns about how to manage the end of life process comes the fear of prosecution in their country of origin. To date, although a handful of British people have been arrested, no relative or friend of the UK citizens who ended their lives in a Swiss Dignitas clinic has been prosecuted under the 1961 Suicide Act.

At Kay Gilderdale's trial in Lewes, the jury was told that her daughter Lynn had discussed the Dignitas option with her mother, but she was in too fragile a state to be moved. After her conviction, Frances Inglis said that she might have considered taking her son Tom there but, in truth, it would not have been a viable option for the Inglis family since Tom had not been in a position to make known his own intentions about his life.

Given the significance of Dignitas, it is necessary to understand its methods, and the motives and experiences of some of the British families who have opted to use its services.

Dignitas was established in 1998 by Ludwig Minelli, a former human rights lawyer. At the time of the Gilderdale and Inglis trials, Minelli gave one visitor a guided tour of his headquarters. As reported, he said, 'There is nothing dramatic about what we do. Our aim is to give the desperate a dignified end to their lives. Dignitas is a not-for-profit organisation which helps people with suicide – in my view the last human right. It is done without risk or pain and in comfortable surroundings.'

The two-storey Dignitas building was situated alongside a machine-parts factory in an industrial estate in the suburb of Pfaffikon. Until the previous year the organisation had operated from a graffiti-covered building in another Zurich suburb, but they had moved when neighbours complained about the number of bodies being carried from the premises.

A staggering five thousand, seven hundred people in sixty-one countries around the world have registered with the group for a fee of two hundred Swiss Francs (about £125 at present rates of exchange), plus an annual fee of eighty-six Swiss francs (about £55). In addition, in order to satisfy Swiss legal requirements for an assisted suicide, a charge of three thousand Swiss francs (£1,875) is levied when the registered individual decides to proceed with their application. This charge covers the preparation of a file for one of Dignitas's six affiliated doctors, who must then decide on the basis of the information contained therein whether they will prescribe the barbiturate for a pain-free death.

By the time the applicant reaches the quiet Swiss suburb, further costs will have brought the grand total to ten and a half thousand Swiss francs (£6,560), unless a 'goodwill reduction' has been negotiated in advance because of lack of funds.

In the back of the building is a space furnished with wooden chairs, and a table topped by a yellow cloth on which stand a candle, a bowl of chocolates and a box of tissues. This is where Dignitas staff, the applicant, and their loved one (or ones) complete the final legal stages of an 'accompaniment'.

Ludwig Minelli explain the procedure: 'We always have two professional companions present at an assisted suicide. First, the bureaucracy is dealt with, including form filling and the presentation of the birth certificate.

'We let the person direct the time, we only direct the technique. Some members tell their whole life story, sharing jokes and memories. No one will hurry them. It's an open procedure which doesn't have to end with a suicide if the person changes their mind.'

The centre has two 'dying rooms'. The larger, with a white leather L-shaped sofa, is the more popular of the two, as friends, family, or both, are generally present. The single bed is covered with a yellow duvet and a window overlooks a small garden.

An anti-vomiting drug, which takes effect after about half an hour, is taken before the barbiturate is administered. In these final tense moments, music is often used to calm both the patient and any family or friends who might be present: a selection of CDs ranging from the Beach Boys to the classical repertoire are stacked by the player. The barbiturate is mixed with water in a plastic cup, ready for the final act. A chocolate is at hand if needed, to mask the taste of the fatal drink.

The vast majority of Dignitas clients are terminally ill or have incurable diseases which are getting progressively worse. After years of such suffering, the clients usually drink the poison in a relaxed and happy frame of mind as death draws close, Minelli said, and spoke of one old Englishwoman who was 'laughing and joking' to the end.

'Members,' Minelli told his visitor, 'usually say goodbye to friends and family, thanking them for their love and support in difficult circumstances. For legal reasons the suicide is videoed, and after death we call the police, who watch the film for proof that the Dignitas member acted alone. Normally there is no complication and the body is either taken to the crematorium or back to the home country.'

In the Dignitas office suite nearby in the building, thirteen part-time staff answer phones or enter details on computers. Minelli, an Anglophile and a devotee of English history, has a portrait of Winston Churchill on the wall.

Inside the differently coloured files is each member's moving personal statement, medical reports, and a final 'Protocol' filled out at the clinic to document their last minutes. In one well-known British case, for example, Minelli indicated that the man involved took the barbiturate at eleven thirty-five a.m., fell asleep four minutes later and passed away at eleven fifty-five a.m.

Minelli has said that he is not troubled by anyone who has made the clear decision to end their life, but is troubled that people are denied the right to an assisted suicide and so recognises the need for the clinic to exist.

At the time of the Gilderdale and Inglis trials there had been no prosecutions in Switzerland following any of the deaths at Dignitas, but Ludwig Minelli was involved in several legal battles to further liberalise the country's law on suicide.

There was a plan by the Swiss authorities to more closely monitor the process the clinic observes but Mr Minelli described the proposals as 'outdated and patronising' pointing out that only twelve out of every hundred applicants to Dignitas are given a green light, adding, 'The rest choose to wait or never get in touch again. People are eased by knowing there is an emergency exit.' This echoes the experiences of those patients in Oregon who have accessed, but not used, a prescription to end their lives at a chosen time.

It is ironic to note that the very existence of the Swiss clinic has allowed several countries to resist liberalising their own laws. Whether intentionally or not, Dignitas has acted as a pressure valve for the issue across Europe.

Mr Minelli had talked in the past of setting up another clinic over the border in Germany, where many of his patients come from, but the legal obstacles were large there, too. At the root of the Swiss government's plans to change the rules was the fear that the country's cheerful ski-and-cuckoo-clock image was being tarnished by the growing reputation that it was a haven for 'suicide tourists'.

Concerned over 'death tourism', right-wing Swiss politicians proposed that groups such as Dignitas should pay large fines – about £30,000 – for helping anyone who had not lived in Zurich for at least a year. A referendum on the proposal might result in a change in the law if it wins the support of more than fifty per cent of electors.

Such a fine – much larger than the existing costs – would probably have to be incorporated into the fee charged to the person ending his or her life and, although it is likely that the number of applications would fall, it would act not as a moral deterrent but merely a fiscal one.

The likelihood that the less well off would be unable to use the service would disappoint the supporters of the clinic's objectives, many of whom, including Mr Minelli himself, have their own experience of losing a loved one to a slow and painful illness.

Minelli's grandmother suffered terribly on her deathbed, at the age of eighty-six. 'She had a kidney problem and endured dreadful pain,' he said. 'I remember my grandmother asking the doctor if he could speed the process. He apologised that it wasn't possible. As a young man I thought, why shouldn't we help people to die, especially when the end is inevitable?'

In one written account he also described the suicide clinic as light-flooded and friendly, with a lovely garden. The letter goes on, 'Beside lies a tiny lake; a little waterfall dabbles, a rill purls flowing to the lake, where goldfishes are swimming. In the background, a garden pavilion and a sunshade.' The letter also urges members to increase their membership fees and 'support our struggle' through donations.

Dignitas needed funds for its campaign to stop the authorities prohibiting organised assisted suicide. Mr Minelli told members that in the new building 'assisted voluntary death proceedings can take place without causing any problems whatsoever. In this respect, you will find some pictures on the reverse side of this information. This certainly is an agreeable information!'

There was, of course, disquiet in many areas over the work that Dignitas, and a smaller Swiss organisation called Ex-International (at a slightly lower cost), carried out. It emerged that record numbers of Britons ended their lives in such Swiss clinics the previous year, as the campaign to decriminalise assisted dying gained ground. Over thirty Britons travelled to die with the help of Dignitas or Ex-International in 2009 as the controversy over assisted death continued.

Baroness Finlay of Llandaff, chairman of the All-Party Parliamentary Group on Dying Well, was quoted as saying the increase in cases was unsurprising given the publicity the issue had received. 'I'm not surprised, because there've been free adverts for Dignitas on the television and radio,' she said.

Lady Finlay, a professor of palliative medicine, said the numbers of Britons ending their lives abroad remained small but raised serious questions. 'How many were terminally ill, how many were depressed, and how were they assessed?' she asked. 'What was the reason behind it – were they made to feel a burden by their family or felt they didn't have a place in society?'

Perhaps by examining some of the cases of those who chose to take that last, short journey, there is an insight to be gained from their experience and that of those who loved them.

Dianne Huff was one such person. For five years her father, John Huff, a former gardener, had struggled against the degenerative condition motor neurone disease (MND), losing first the use of his arms, then his speech and mobility. Once physically fit and active, he now faced a future where he would lose control completely over his physical movements and require constant care – a healthy mind trapped in a ravaged, non-functioning body.

He had first decided on Dignitas four years earlier. His wife, Barbara, had hoped that her husband would have a change of heart, but he feared that he would become too ill to travel to Switzerland. Swiss law demands that the person who has chosen to end his or her life has to administer the drug themselves. As motor neurone disease affects the ability to move and swallow, it had been a race against time.

Also contributing to Mr Huff's decision to approach Dignitas was his fear that his family would be at risk should they want to help him end his life in the UK. Already unable to write, he had asked for his daughter's help in filling out the application. Once a date at the clinic was provided, his friends and family were able to gather at the Huff home to say their goodbyes.

John Huff's family accompanied him on his momentous trip in August 2006. In Zurich, on the last night of his life, they shared drinks and dinner together for the last time. Dianne, his daughter, later told of her father's big, fond smile and loud laughter, even though the whole family knew what lay ahead of them in the morning.

That evening, as they sat at a riverside restaurant before returning to their hotel, it must have seemed to the family a terrible parody of the life they would have shared if Mr Huff had not been struck down with his illness. Now, even drinking his gin and tonic (through a straw) brought a grimace because his taste buds had been irrevocably changed by motor neurone disease; there seemed no respite from the changes it had wrought.

Nevertheless, John Huff remained cheerful and relaxed: he felt he had a measure of control over his illness, and he was not in a hospice unable to communicate his needs as he had always feared he might be. The relief had been palpable every since the family had touched down in Zurich.

On the final day, the Huff family arrived at the Dignitas

offices and were shown to the flat. Small, neat, simply furnished, and hundreds of miles from their home in south London, it was the last place that the family had ever previously imagined they would find themselves. Now they were very grateful that it existed.

After the anti-sickness drug was administered to Mr Huff, it was time to prepare the barbiturate. When mixed, the solution is cloudy; when it turns clear it is ready for consumption. John spoke little but his mood remained upbeat. Barbara took him to the bathroom to ask once more if he were sure that he wanted to end his life. She knew that her husband had been told that he could be expected to live for only six more months, and although she hoped that he would choose to endure those last few months, she also understood when he told her that yes, he was ready to die.

His daughters helped him onto the bed, then stood aside to allow the video camera to record Mr Huff accepting the barbiturate, which he drank through a straw. He then lay down to sleep. Within half an hour he was pronounced dead.

The family felt their loss deeply, but they also had some measure of relief from seeing how peaceful Mr Huff looked. The journey home was much harder for them than the journey out. They had booked a return ticket in case he changed his mind, but now his seat on the plane remained empty.

*

Richard Geary was another who suffered the pain and consequences of watching a loved one battle a crippling illness. In this case the disease was Multiple System Atrophy (MSA), a degenerative neurological disorder, and the victim his wife, Jenny, to whom he was married for over forty years.

Slowly, Jenny's ability to walk and to coordinate her movements was stripped away. The loss of her ability to read was a great blow to Jenny, and it was a constant source of grief to Richard to see his once vibrant wife now trapped in a chair, her body inexorably shutting down on her. Towards the end of her life, Richard had to shower, dress and spoon-feed his wife. She began to find it difficult to talk, and it was apparent that the illness would soon start to attack her ability to swallow.

Jenny chose to fly to Zurich. She had lost her father after a long illness and Richard had watched his own mother die of leukaemia. Jenny made the decision that she did not wish to endure a protracted death, she already felt that she had been robbed of so much: the loss of interaction with her children, grandchildren and friends; being unable to care for her two ponies . . . she wondered whether, if the animals she loved were so desperately ill, would a vet hesitate to 'put them out of their misery'.

In August 2009, just as the DPP, Keir Starmer, released

his guidelines on prosecution in cases of assisted deaths, Jenny Geary, by then aged sixty-one, flew to Switzerland. The doctor at Dignitas observed that she had arrived only just in time as, within weeks, the disease would have prevented her from swallowing the 50ml of barbiturate necessary to end her life.

Once Jenny had made up her mind to end her life, she was relieved to have the support of her family and friends. Nevertheless, her son and daughter found it difficult and painful to accept her decision. Even though they were adults with families of their own, the thought of life without their mother was painful to contemplate. But they also recognised that if she was in control of how and when her life would end, it would be an important part of allowing her to cope with the last months of her illness.

Asked later how he felt once his wife had died, Richard said, 'A bit of guilt in a way . . . but at the front of my mind all the time was that the end result would have been far worse – of being kept alive artificially until she'd contracted pneumonia and died – had we not chosen this course of action.'

Richard Geary would not have changed the course of action he and his wife took, but he subsequently added his voice to the chorus of the many who wish that a facility such as Dignitas existed in the UK. When he returned to his home in Cornwall, he walked into his local police station at Saltash and told them what had happened. Later he had to make a statement to detectives and a report went to the Crown Prosecution Service, but he heard nothing as to whether he would be prosecuted as the months passed.

Like Sir Terry Pratchett, Richard is in favour of an independent panel to assess the right to die on a case-by-case basis and would like to see a facility like that of Dignitas open in the UK. It cost his family close to £9,000 to make all the arrangements Jenny needed, and he is aware that not all families can afford such a price.

There is still disquiet about the possibility of a 'death clinic' opening in the UK, and controversy intensified with the death of Craig Ewert. His was one of the most high profile of the Dignitas deaths, and it could hardly have been anything else, given that it was filmed and shown on television.

A fifty-nine-year-old retired university professor and father of two, Mr Ewert was shown turning off his ventilator and taking a lethal dose of drugs washed down with apple juice. Mary, his wife of thirty-seven years, sat and talked with him until he passed away.

This was the first time an assisted suicide was shown on British television and it was condemned as dangerous and grotesque by those who feared that it would 'undermine people's right to life' and risked glorifying suicide. Others, however, praised it as a valuable contribution to the ongoing debate.

Mr Ewert, an American who had been living in Harrogate, North Yorkshire, was diagnosed with motor neurone disease five months before his death. His health deteriorated rapidly. He required a ventilator to help him breathe, and the chronic wasting disease threatened to rob him of his ability to swallow.

Mr Ewert paid Dignitas £3000 to help him end his life. Oscar-winning documentary director John Zaritsky was given access to Dignitas and, with the approval of Craig Ewert and his family, recorded everything that happened on 26 September 2006 and the film was shown in a number of countries.

In the film, he talked lucidly about the reasons for his decision to die, and described his body as a 'living tomb'. Again, evidence had to be prepared to show that in taking his life, Mr Ewert acted alone and so he was recorded using his teeth to activate a timer to switch off his life support machine.

With Beethoven's Ninth Symphony playing in the background, Craig Ewert drank the lethal dose of sodium phenobarbital from a cup, using a straw to do so. Mr Bernhard, the Dignitas escort who held the cup for him, said, 'I wish you good travelling.' With his wife holding his hand, he lost consciousness minutes later.

Later, after a loud beep announced that the ventilator had turned itself off, his escort checked the pulse in Mr Ewert's neck and said, 'He's gone.' Mrs Ewert was then seen kissing her husband's body.

Mr Ewert died but in truth, this was about a great deal more than a desire to cease living. Like many with an illness that would lead to an inexorable decline, Mr Ewert had faced a stark dilemma. Although he still felt that he wanted to live, he was no longer certain that he could be in control of his physical decline and feared missing the point at which he was still able to act to end his life – without the intervention of another's hand.

He said: 'I cannot take the risk. Let's face it, when you're completely paralysed and cannot talk, how do you let somebody know you are suffering? This could be a complete and utter hell. Once I become completely paralysed then I am nothing more than a living tomb that takes in nutrients through a tube in the stomach – it's painful.'

Craig Ewert decided not to allow his children, Ivan and Katrina, aged thirty-five and thirty-three respectively, to be at his deathbed in Zurich because he feared it would make it more difficult for him to go through with it.

Director Zaritsky wanted the film to be controversial, to spark a public debate. He said, 'That was probably the most difficult moment of my entire career. To film a man dying that you had followed for four days was pretty amazing. Craig was the hero of the film.'

There was no shortage of public reaction to the film, as reported in the media. Dominica Roberts of the Pro-Life Alliance said it was 'both sad and dangerous to show this kind of thing on the television. It is sad because any suicide is sad. It is dangerous because it could have a copycat effect. The point of the laws [is] to protect vulnerable people.'

Dr Trevor Stammers of the Christian Medical Fellowship considered the spectacle of having your death broadcast on TV grotesque, and Phyllis Bowman of Right to Life, believed it was 'promoting assisted suicide. What kind of effect do they imagine it is going to have on a depressive? It undermines the vulnerable and it also undermines people's right to life.'

Phil Willis, the Lib-Dem MP for Harrogate and Knaresborough, where Mr Ewert lived, said, 'The idea that we can make a documentary actually in some ways glorifying suicide seems to me to be a step we should at least challenge in terms of the morality of it, if not condemn.'

Barbara Gibbon of Sky Real Lives, however, said: 'This is an issue that more and more people are confronting and this documentary is an informative, articulate and educated insight into the decisions some people have to make. I think it's important that TV broadcasters can stimulate debate about this issue.'

Mary Ewert said her husband believed he had two choices: to die, or to suffer and die. His fifty-nine-year-old widow defended her husband's decision: 'He felt he couldn't be certain that he'd go through with it, and he said that until the morning we were in the Dignitas apartment. He knew that at any point he could decide not to go through with it.

'Craig talks at length about all of this, about his situation being one where his choice is between death and suffering and death. Death, perhaps sooner than he would have chosen, was the logical choice.' Mary also defended the documentary. 'Craig was keen to have it shown,' she said, 'because when death is hidden and private, people don't face their fears.'

Craig's son Ivan said, 'I am very proud of what Dad did. He always talked about it and when the time comes to make that decision, I am sure I will be able to do so too.

'I intend to become a fee-paying member of Dignitas as I age, so I will be able to choose when I am ready. His mind was still very clear, he was still eloquent, but his body was a living tomb. He told me he would prefer to die.'

According to a poll taken soon after the programme was aired, more than two thirds of people would back a change in the law on assisted suicide.

The survey, carried out by YouGov for the *Sunday Times*, also concluded that sixty-one per cent would consider ending their life if they were suffering from a terminal disease. YouGov surveyed more than two thousand members of the public online; sixty-nine per cent supported changing legislation to offer immunity from prosecution to people who help friends and relatives travel to foreign clinics to commit suicide. More than sixty per cent of those surveyed said Sky was right to broadcast the documentary.

Believing that you would end your life, should you one day find that you are diagnosed with a terminal or degenerative disease, does not mean however that you will act on that conviction.

In 2006 writer Charlotte Raven found out that she had the incurable degenerative disorder Huntington's Disease. It is a brain condition that causes the progressive loss of control over movement and of mental faculties. Only one year earlier, she had found out that her father had the disease and was offered the test to find out if she had inherited the condition.

Such tests, of course, are becoming more readily available. It can be argued that the availability of such tests has been driven not only by medical advances in gene technology but in a demand for greater knowledge and control over our health.

The diagnosis proved devastating for Raven. Her daughter was only eighteen months old, yet her first instinct was to end her life before her physical degeneration became too advanced. She wrote, 'My first suicidal thought was a kind of epiphany – like Batman figuring out his escape from the Joker's death trap.'

One in four of those who develop the condition do attempt to end their lives. Raven wondered why three-quarters decide not to die, as she believed that to be reduced to a state where she would require constant nursing would be degrading and anathema to the way that she had always lived.

It took a trip to Venezuela to a village called Barranquitas – where a series of genetic flaws has led to a disproportionately high number of people suffering with Huntington's – to challenge her long-held assumptions. There she found an acceptance of the disease and the realisation that not all 'sufferers' are stripped of their humanity in the way that she had imagined.

It made Raven question the way that people in the affluent West are being 'sold' the idea of an 'easeful death', shifting suicide into the arena of an idea rather than acknowledging it as a physical process. She left Venezuela no longer viewing suicide as a form of self-deliverance but as a destructive and 'immodest' act.

Her change of mind was a relief to her husband, who had opposed her decision to end her life prematurely. She wrote, 'Registering the discomfort of existence, I felt a great wave of self-pity, the first since my diagnosis. I felt worthy of being cherished and knew I'd do whatever it took to survive.

'Back home, I told my husband he was right. The case for carrying on can't be argued. Suicide is rhetoric. Life is life.'

Though not all who suffer choose to end their lives, it is those who do that seem to drive the debate.

In the summer of 2008 a letter appeared in the *Sun*:

I escorted my partner of 28 years, Raymond Cutkelvin, to Dignitas last year to assist him on his final journey after he was diagnosed with pancreatic cancer. All staff treated us BOTH with care, respect and compassion and were extremely professional, giving invaluable support and advice at all times.

Raymond was very intelligent and of sound mind when he decided to end his life. It was a beautiful ending for a beautiful person, which should have taken place in the UK.

The right to die is the last human right.

The letter was signed Alan Cutkelvin Rees, and shortly after its publication Raymond's full story emerged. Raymond Cutkelvin, accompanied by Alan, had chosen to die at the Dignitas clinic a year earlier, after paying a fee of £4,500.

Alan, outraged that Raymond had to die 'in exile', decided to talk about the events leading up to his partner's death in an effort to force the Government to clarify the law on assisted suicide. He was adamant that even though his actions in helping Raymond were illegal in the UK, he was content to face arrest. Like many who are forced to watch a loved one suffer, he chose to listen to his partner's wish to die with dignity.

Tests in August 2006 had revealed a large tumour in Raymond's pancreas and doctors said that they were unable to operate. He had treatment at the Whittington Hospital in north London but, in light of the aggressive nature of his illness, chose not to have chemotherapy and began to research euthanasia sites on the internet.

The couple had been together for twenty-eight years and in November 2006 took part in a civil partnership ceremony. When the time came to leave for Switzerland, they flew to Zurich with Raymond's niece, a friend, and euthanasia campaigner Dr Michael Irwin.

Raymond's last evening was difficult; it was a struggle for him to keep his pain at bay even with the morphine he was taking. The night was fraught, too, with Alan also having to come to terms with the fact that the next day would be the last that he and Raymond would spend together.

In the morning, the group went to the clinic. With all paperwork completed and final checks made as to Raymond's state of mind and intentions, like the many before him he took medication to prevent nausea before taking the dose of barbiturates.

With his favourite music playing, Raymond danced with his niece and hugged Alan goodbye. He lay down to sleep and Alan repeated 'I love you, Raymond' until his partner died.

Raymond's ashes were flown back to the UK and were interred in his family's plot in Edinburgh. Alan, like many carers, had given up working for the duration of his partner's illness and had to apply for help with the cost of the funeral. A state benefit does exist for this purpose, but staff at the Department of Work and Pensions had never had to deal with a burial of an assisted suicide. Like many in the UK, they were in uncharted territory and unsure at first how best to proceed.

Alan, still grieving, remained clear about his actions and has said of Raymond's death, 'I loved him and could not allow him to suffer. To me, it would have been an act of kindness and compassion.'

Over two years after Raymond Cutkelvin's death, Alan Cutkelvin Rees was arrested and questioned in connection with the assisted suicide. He spoke publicly of the events as details of the DPP's new guidelines were released – one of the key changes being the removal of the factor that considered whether the person assisting was a family member.

He said, 'It's good news and certainly a step forward, but there's still a long way to go. It has made things clearer for people who are considering assisted suicide. And for their relatives and friends, because it's not just a case of going with a loved one to Switzerland, it's facing whatever one might have to face after returning to the UK.

'This is an extremely sensitive and important subject which needs further discussion by politicians, the Church, and people like myself who have been through it. At least now the door is open and the matter hasn't been swept under the carpet.'

For anybody, having the prospect of prosecution hanging over them is very difficult. Alan was confident, though, that a jury would understand his actions and motivations.

A similar story was told by Dave Richards, diagnosed at fifty-seven with Huntington's Disease. Four years later he hadn't in fact suffered any mental deterioration but his speech had become faint and he had difficulty swallowing.

As he prepared to fly to Dignitas, Mr Richards, who had travelled alone by taxi from his home on the Isle of Wight, gave an interview over a meal in his room at the Gatwick Hilton. He preferred to dine in his room rather than in the hotel restaurant because he was concerned about causing public discomfort with the involuntary movements of his arms and legs. Over dinner, he declined offers of help, preferring to eat his bread roll dry since he was unable to butter it.

He revealed that he had lost the strength in his legs. After a fall the previous year he feared that if he waited much longer he might not be physically capable of making the journey to Zurich.

The concerns that drove his decision to end his life reflected the concerns of others who have applied to Dignitas: fear that he would be confined to an institution, that he would become entirely dependent on others to care for him, that he would be unable to swallow and would be fed through a tube. Above all, he feared the prospect that he would be kept alive indefinitely in what to him appeared as an intolerable condition.

Dave Richards wished that he could have arranged to die on the Isle of Wight, but it was not an option. No matter that his GP, his neurologist, his psychologist and his care worker knew of his intention to end his life and had all wished him well.

Dr Michael Irwin accompanied Mr Richards on the flight. He later spoke of what happened in Zurich. After they arrived, 'We got to the hotel and spent four or five hours just talking. We discussed everything from Fred Hoyle and is there life in the universe apart from ourselves, to Formula One racing.'

At the Dignitas clinic, Mr Richards was helped onto a bed, where he sat and took the lethal medication. To comply with Swiss law, Dr Irwin informed the police of the events he witnessed. He said, 'The policeman questioned me about how we arrived and where we stayed the previous night. After another half an hour I was told I could leave.

'You have got to be very determined to go to Dignitas and the escort has got to be strong-minded. Am I breaking the law? The police cannot tell me. Other people helped Dave with the paperwork. Various people would have played a part in breaking the law.'

The Dignitas deaths are not always solitary affairs. Some married couples have arranged to end their lives together at the clinic.

In February 2009, Peter Duff, aged eighty, and his

seventy-year-old wife Penelope, both ill with terminal cancer, told friends they were leaving their two million-pound house in Bath and moving to a second home in Dorset. In reality, they were making the journey to Dignitas to end their lives together in an assisted suicide pact.

After they had died, a statement released by their daughter said, simply, 'Peter and Penny Duff passed away peacefully together in Zurich after a long battle against their terminal cancer.

'Penny had fought a rare cancer since 1992 and Peter's colon cancer had spread to his liver. Their decision in no way reflected on the wonderful and humbling care they received from their consultant, doctors and nurses, for which the family, and they, were so appreciative.'

Mrs Duff, it emerged, had suffered from GIST, a rare form of cancer found in the digestive system, most often in the wall of the stomach. Her husband had cared for her until he became too ill himself to do so. It is a poignant circumstance that a couple, who have dedicated their lives to one another, choose to die together because of terminal illness.

The Duffs were not the only couple to come to the attention of the outside world because of the decision they reached. A more high-profile joint journey to Dignitas took place in July 2009 when the internationally renowned classical music conductor, Sir Edward Downes, and his wife also travelled to Zurich because they wished to end their lives.

Sir Edward, eighty-five, was by then virtually blind and had suffered loss of hearing, while seventy-four-year-old Lady Downes, a former ballet dancer and choreographer, had cancer.

The couple's decision was supported by their forty-one-year old son, Caractacus, and their daughter, Boudicca, aged thirty-nine (both named after leaders who had revolted against Roman rule), who were at their parents' bedside as they died.

Caractacus Downes said afterwards, 'It was very calm and very simple. The actual final draught is a small glass of clear liquid. They both drank that and lay down on the bed and were both asleep in a couple of minutes. It was very sad but we were content that they had been given the opportunity to end their lives in the way they wanted to.'

The son and daughter were interviewed by the police under caution, although there was no suggestion of any suspicious behaviour on their part.

Mr Downes said his parents decided to go to Switzerland when they did because they were worried that his mother's health would deteriorate and prevent her from travelling.

Boudicca Downes said, 'I am absolutely for the way my parents died and I hope things change in England. I believe in choice and I believe things should change.'

*

Not all couples who arrive at the same decision can expect understanding. One couple whose deaths caused controversy were Robert and Jennifer Stokes, aged fifty-nine and fifty-three respectively. Neither of them, a UK inquest was to hear, was terminally ill. They both had a history of mental illness and failed suicide attempts and, while both were said to be in constant pain from disability and various chronic illnesses, these conditions were not severe to the point of being considered life-threatening.

Dignitas, however, agreed to the joint suicide of Robert and Jennifer, and the couple died at the clinic, in each other's arms, in March 2003.

The Stokes case raised serious and disquieting concerns about 'suicide tourism' and the manner in which Dignitas helped people. Under Swiss law, assisted suicide was only a crime if those providing the help could be shown to have acted out of self-interest. But patients must have a terminal illness and be of sound judgement, neither of which applied to this couple.

The year after their deaths, David Morris, the Bedfordshire coroner, said, 'No evidence has been put to me that either of them was in any terminal state or expected imminent death.'

This evidence marked a notable departure from the core facts pertaining to the other British individuals who had chosen to end their days at Dignitas.

The couple had first met in the 1970s when they were

both patients at a psychiatric hospital. Jennifer Stokes had a history of depression and had made several attempts to end her life. She was believed to have been suffering from paranoia.

In 1983, a road accident left her in constant pain from severe spinal problems that proved inoperable. She frequently needed help washing and dressing and her health deteriorated further in 1998 after she was diagnosed with diabetes.

Her husband Robert had epilepsy and could have up to three severe fits each week. Like his wife, he also had a history of depression and had also been plagued by suicidal tendencies.

Although the couple's lives were difficult and not without issues of pain, it took their son, David, to articulate what was so unsettling about their case. He said, 'I know my parents were not terminally ill. The only terminal illness they had was in their heads.'

The couple had made previous attempts to end their lives, once in 1990 and again in 2001. On both occasions they had been found and rushed to hospital. Friends did acknowledge that the couple feared becoming separated and placed in different care homes, and no doubt such concerns were part of what influenced their decision.

Dignitas had come to the Stokes's attention after the case of Reginald Crew, the first British man to die at the clinic, became news. By the time that the couple were in a care home in Leighton Buzzard, Bedfordshire, they discussed once more how they might manage their own deaths, and made their plans accordingly.

They wrote to their solicitor detailing arrangements for the repatriation of their bodies and their funeral wishes and simply left their care home one morning and flew to Zurich.

The case caused a furore in Switzerland. The Swiss authorities held an inquiry, the outcome of which led to proposals to tighten regulations surrounding the administration of assisted suicide cases.

Once the inquest on the Stokes's deaths was concluded, their daughter Helen said, 'Although I cannot condone Dignitas's actions I do accept and understand my parents' decision. They both suffered many years of ill health, and the possibility of their lives continuing without each other was an unbearable thought. I do believe that it was with fear and courage that my parents chose to take their own lives.'

These are just a handful of the many cases which have fuelled the arguments as to the rights and wrongs of allowing or assisting in the death of someone close. Like the Gilderdales and the Inglises, families involved at the epicentre of the debate will rarely find a clear and unequivocal agreement between all involved during such emotionally draining events.

It is right that society takes into account the families of those caught up in assisted suicide, but they can only ever be part of the picture. Their views of the issue will understandably be dictated by their own often troubled experiences. It will also take a more dispassionate analysis by professionals and those outside the immediate family circle, to shape the future direction of our ethical understanding and legal framework.

In July 2009 the British Medical Association annual conference rejected a bid to change the law on prosecuting relatives who accompany patients to suicide clinics. By a narrow margin – fifty-two to forty-four percent – BMA members voted down proposals for lifting the threat of police investigations into those accompanying a patient at an assisted death. Doctors rejected calls to exempt relatives and/or friends from criminal prosecution.

Their decision came just a week before the House of Lords was to discuss the matter. An amendment by Lord Falconer was asking for legal protection to relatives who travel abroad to assisted suicide clinics such as Dignitas. The peer's initiative had won the support of Sir Terry Pratchett.

Doctors at the BMA conference also turned down, by a larger margin, another motion calling for legislation to allow patients who are 'terminally ill and have mental capacity' to choose an assisted death. The BMA had switched position on assisted deaths several times but had supported the current legal status since 2006.

Dr Kailash Chand told the BMA conference in

Liverpool that it was a matter of enabling patients to die with dignity. 'If the physical pain is unbearable,' he said, 'we must not put [legal] pressure on loved ones who want to travel abroad to assist suicides.

'If enforced, more than a hundred people would by now have been prosecuted. This situation leaves physicians unprotected. The fear of prosecution hangs over the heads of all concerned.'

But Professor Baroness Finlay of Llandaff, chair of the All-Party parliamentary group on dying well, urged doctors to resist any change. 'The current law works well,' she told the conference. 'It has a stern face and a kind heart. The stern face deters coercion. The current law works on a case-by-case basis. As it stands, it is compassionate. Is there a problem?'

A London doctor, Jackie Davis, asked the conference whether patients should not have the right to choose, 'even if we do not approve of their choice. Do we have the right to deny them the ultimate patient choice?'

The BMA vote followed a recent survey of doctors that found two-thirds remained opposed to assisted deaths. Many doctors privately admitted that, at some future point, they might consider taking their own lives but were worried about the responsibility of becoming involved in such decisions relating to their patients.

The heads of different religions also held strong views, and three of them joined forces to stop a Lords' amendment that they feared would pave the way to legalising euthanasia.

Dr Rowan Williams, the Archbishop of Canterbury; Vincent Nichols, the Archbishop of Westminster, and the Chief Rabbi, Sir Jonathan Sacks, urged the peers to reject proposals that would allow families to help their loved ones die abroad without the threat of prosecution. In a joint letter to the *Daily Telegraph*, they wrote that such a legal change 'would surely put vulnerable people at serious risk, especially sick people who are anxious about the burden their illness may be placing on others.'

It was the first time since his appointment to the post that the new Catholic Archbishop of Westminster had openly joined with the head of the Anglican Church and the Chief Rabbi to intervene in a legislative matter. In their letter, the clerics also criticised legislators for trying to legalise euthanasia by the back door. 'This amendment,' they wrote, 'would mark a shift in British law towards legalising euthanasia. We do not believe that such a fundamental change in the law should be sought by way of an amendment to an already complex Bill.'

As has been demonstrated by the differing opinions on the issue, the dilemma of how to cope and react to a loved one's illness or disability affects not just mothers, but every member of a family and a circle of close friends, regardless of age and social status.

The cases of Kay Gilderdale and Frances Inglis were still being debated when the veteran broadcaster Ray Gosling announced on a television documentary that he had ended the life of a man who was dying from complications that had arisen from HIV/AIDS.

The programme in which Gosling revealed this news was a local edition of the BBC's regional documentary series *Inside Out*. The fifteen-minute long segment featured the presenter reflecting, mainly in a light-hearted manner, on his own mortality, and 'exploring the choices we make at the end of our lives.'

Amidst talking about different types of coffin or the selection of funeral music, the seventy-year-old Gosling suddenly changed gear to make what he called 'my own rather startling confession' while strolling through a graveyard.

'Maybe this is the time to share a secret that I've kept for quite a long time? I killed someone once. He was a young chap who had been my lover and he got Aids . . . and he was in terrible pain. I took a pillow and I smothered him.'

It was an extraordinary statement and Gosling found himself at the centre of a media storm. He was questioned by the police and was initially arrested on suspicion of murder in February 2010. Yet by September of that year, Gosling was charged with wasting police time after the Crown Prosecution Service decided there was enough evidence to 'provide a realistic prospect of proving that Mr Gosling's confession was false'.

Speaking outside the court that September, Gosling admitted that he had not killed his lover and said: 'I was not even in the country when he died, but I would have done it.' It was a remarkable turn of events and the facts, once they emerged, seemed to underline the potential for passions to run high over the issue of assisted suicide. And in some, it can even create an emotional firestorm.

13

The Shadow of Death

There was no shortage of opinion about the cases of Kay Gilderdale and Frances Inglis. Sympathy for the plight of the two mothers was almost universal, as was criticism of the different outcomes of their trials.

While Kay walked away from court a free woman, Frances began a life sentence and the court rang out with cries of 'Shame on You!' as the judge made his recommendation that she serve nine years behind bars. There was, too, widespread feeling that, having suffered so much, neither woman should have been prosecuted in the first place.

The jury had taken less than two hours to decide that Kay Gilderdale was not guilty as charged, and the judge questioning why the case had ever been put to a jury highlighted the public mood of support for Kay.

In the period leading up to her trial at Lewes Crown Court, Kay had co-operated with the BBC's *Panorama* programme. Shown some days after the verdict, the programme revealed some of her own feelings as she talked to Jeremy Vine about the events that had led her to court.

Kay, quietly spoken as ever, was clear that if she again had to face the choice as to whether or not she should help Lynn, she would do so regardless of the consequences.

Listening to her recount Lynn's last hours was compelling. Kay had seen absolute determination in her daughter's face, the kind of look that she remembered from when Lynn was young. She had set her mind on an escape from the body that had for too long failed her, and had too long imprisoned her.

Kay's words were unbearably moving. She said, 'You are torn apart because you have one part of you that is wanting to respect your daughter's wishes, and you've got your heart being ripped out at the same time because all you want to do is to make them better and keep them alive.'

Despite everything, every medical effort, the many years of careful nursing at home and the love, tenderness, patience and devotion, Kay and Richard had failed. They had not made her better. Now their wish to keep her alive perhaps served only their desperate need not to be without her. The family had thought about Dignitas but knew that moving Lynn would probably have caused her broken bones and more pain.

Kay described how she had to listen as her daughter pleaded for her help, begged her to get more morphine to ensure that she could end her life. It was a cold December night, the quiet outside the house belying the turmoil within, where mother and daughter had shared a lifetime together.

December being a time when families are making arrangements for the Christmas holidays, Kay was expecting her son Steven and his wife Sarah to come and visit with their two young children. Perhaps Lynn, who loved the children, would wait until after Christmas at least . . . ?

But no, Lynn did not waver. She knew that for her mother there would never be a 'good' or 'better' or 'right' time to lose her daughter.

What should Kay do for 'the best'? Listen to her daughter or refuse to help. She thought of the many, many times that Lynn had said, 'Mum, you know I don't want to be here. You can't fix me any more.'

Kay tried to talk to her once more, to persuade her to carry on, but it was of no use. Every fibre in her daughter's being strained towards focusing on ending her suffering. This was not about losing hope – hope had sustained Lynn and her loved ones for so many long years – this was different and distinct. Lynn was clear-headed in her assessment that, for her, hope had gone. There would be no recovery. What she needed now was release.

Kay left the room and went to get the morphine.

Lynn asked to say goodbye to the family cats Willow and Shadow. Only Willow could be found and brought to Lynn to stroke for the last time. Shadow was nowhere to be seen.

With the syringes to hand, Lynn refused to let her mother come close to her. For Kay, the instinct to help her daughter was hard to suppress and, as Lynn struggled to lift the Hickman line, Kay reached over to help her. But Lynn, who had long ago researched the implications of a loved one assisting suicide, pushed her away: she knew that she had to administer the drugs herself or her mother would risk criminal charges.

Lynn said something – and the word 'frightened'. Kay was sure she meant of facing the unknown, of what would become of her after she died, but Lynn said, no, she was frightened what would happen to her mother and frightened that the attempt to end her life would fail.

Lynn connected the two syringes to the inlet tubes of the Hickman line and put a hand over each. In the most extraordinary moment, as Lynn held the plungers of the syringes, the lights in the house cut out. A circuit had blown, but for that moment it was as if the house itself felt the night's upheaval and sorrow.

As Lynn depressed the last plunger, Kay said, 'Wait!' But Lynn looked steadily at her mother and shook her head. As the morphine entered her bloodstream, she lost consciousness.

It was not a seamless death. Lynn's resistance to the drug was such that despite the massive dose – 630 milligrams – of morphine, her shattered body continued to function.

At three-thirty in the morning she woke for a brief few moments and gave her mother a loving look before falling unconscious again. She would not have doubted that Kay would be there. And indeed Kay did not leave Lynn's side for twenty-four hours. She talked to her, held her hand and stroked her face, hoping that her daughter could still hear her, trusting that Lynn's determination was such that she did not fear what was happening to her.

Kay stayed vigilant lest Lynn start to show signs of distress and determined to be with her at the end. Just as she had delivered her daughter into this world, so she would be there to ease her departure from it.

After three hours, Lynn's breathing became more laboured. Kay listened as it grew worse and it was at this point that she decided she would crush up some of Lynn's sedatives and give them to her via her nasal tube. It was a crucial decision, not only for her daughter but for herself; a decision that would radically alter the course of how she would be regarded in the eyes of the law.

It was simple enough to take some of Lynn's sleeping tablets, crush them with a pestle and mortar to turn them into powder, dissolve the powder in some water, and then put the solution in the tube. Kay was adept at feeding her daughter, whether with nutrients or medication, and had done so with dedication over seventeen long years. Legally, however, her actions that night left her exposed to a charge of attempted murder.

The prosecution would later argue that, in administering the powdered sedatives, Kay was killing Lynn. It was a charge that Kay, or anyone who knew her, would never accept but, sitting beside her daughter and hearing her struggling to breathe, Kay felt compelled to act to help Lynn to die.

Lynn's pain relief seemed to be wearing off despite the high quantity of morphine that she had taken.

Kay was exhausted and emotionally wrung out and what followed next is unclear. At one stage it was believed that Kay administered the anti-depressant Sertraline because she later said as much to Lynn's GP, but no trace of it was found in Lynn's system. It would also be claimed that Kay injected Lynn with air in an attempt to cause an embolism, but Kay had no recollection of having done so. Neither could she remember being on the phone to Exit, although she did recall rushing frantically from Lynn's room to her own computer to search for help on the internet. She didn't want to leave Lynn's side but was desperate not to let her down.

From a legal point of view, these actions were part of a process that Lynn did not control, but when asked about her intervention, Kay said, 'Yes, but I felt that Lynn was dying after the morphine overdose. She started to show signs of stress with her breathing. I was really worried that she was suffering in some way, so I got a few tablets – again, not the cocktail that the papers reported or the prosecution made it sound to be. I crushed them and I gave them to her.'

When Kay called Exit it was because she wanted to make sure that her daughter's death would be comfortable. The pain that had defined her young life should not accompany her to the bitter end.

Those twenty-four hours were almost too difficult to bear. The spectre that Lynn might not die was one frightening scenario, but there were others that, in Lynn's eyes, were far worse: she could, for example, suffer acute liver or brain damage and be placed on life-support machinery, away from her mother's loving care . . .

And Kay was alone. Alone with her thoughts in turmoil, mechanically obeying her daughter's wishes while her heart was crying out for Lynn to stay. 'I didn't want her to go,' Kay said. 'I wanted to call for help. I wanted my son Steve there. I wanted Lynn's father, Richard, there. I wanted her to find peace.

'I had been crying solidly all that time. I thought I was acting OK, but when I look back I see the longer I went without sleep and food, the more distressed I became.'

Here was a mother who had been through hell and back, and was now being forced to walk through hell again, without the support of those who had been there for her over the long years and who loved Lynn as much as she did. Then, at seven in the morning on 4 December, Lynn's breathing suddenly stopped. She was finally at peace, but it was at this moment that her mother collapsed, exhausted from the physical and emotional demands of the last day and night.

When she was at last able to compose herself, Kay picked

up her mobile phone. In the day and the hours leading up to Lynn's death, her father, Richard, had sent several texts to ask how his daughter was, just as he always did. Kay had resisted saying any more in her replies other than that Lynn was sleeping; she didn't want to risk incriminating Richard in what was happening at the house.

Even though the couple's marriage had ended some six years earlier and Richard had now remarried, he and Kay remained good friends and were both devoted to helping their daughter with her struggle. Now, Kay simply sent a text to Richard asking him to come to the house. In his heart he knew that an end had been reached, that his beautiful daughter had gone.

He drove to the house they had once all shared and as he walked into Lynn's bedroom it was as if all the years of sorrow he had felt weighed down on him. It was over.

As an ex-police sergeant, Richard knew the formalities of what had to happen next. The police would be called, and a doctor. Kay was shattered, she had nothing left to give. When she had begun to nurse Lynn she was a woman of thirty-seven; now she was fifty-four years old and facing the prospect of a murder enquiry and the full glare of public scrutiny.

Those last few painful, traumatic and private hours with Lynn would now be picked over by investigators and the media. Kay did not wish to become a test case for mercy killing or assisted suicide, and yet that was what would happen. Her case was to become a byword, a touchstone, for the emotions of a nation and the divided rulings of the police, the Crown Prosecution Service and the Judiciary.

Kay's family believed that her admission that she helped Lynn would be the focus of the prosecution. Although Lynn's postmortem revealed that she had died from morphine toxicity, it was unable to establish whether it was the morphine that she had administered herself or the dose that her mother had given her that had caused her death. It would emerge that it was only this lack of clarity that saved Kay from the more serious charge of murder.

As it stood, Kay was charged with attempted murder and the wheels were set in motion. The Gilderdales were shocked and, for Kay, the shock turned to anger that the authorities could believe that she would at any stage want to kill the daughter she had cherished for so long.

The law was a safeguard for the vulnerable, but when it came to a case like Lynn's, that same law jeopardised the lives of those who loved and cared for her, and had prevented her managing her death as she would have wished. If it had not been for the law, Lynn would not have had to fear for her mother's future, and she could have asked her beloved father and brother to be present while she was dying. Together, without the fear of failure or prosecution, they could have said goodbye. Lynn would have been able to tell her family that she loved them and then found the peace she so desperately sought, but that had been denied her.

The family could have supported one another in this painful situation; instead, Kay was left alone, frantically attempting to cope and to monitor her daughter's efforts to die, and now she faced a possible prison sentence.

In the end, Kay was found not guilty and the judge, Mr Justice Bean, praised the jury and took the rare step of criticising the Crown Prosecution Service for rejecting Kay's plea that she was guilty of assisting her daughter's death and bringing her case to trial.

It is worth looking at what Mr Justice Bean said when he addressed the jury: 'I do not normally comment on the verdicts of juries but in this case their decision ... shows that common sense, decency and humanity which makes jury trials so important in a case of this kind.'

The law has often been described as sometimes acting as 'a hammer to crack a nut', it is thought of as too unwieldy, too arcane, too slow moving and too restricted. In a case such as Kay's, it is revealed in a better light.

There can be no hard and fast rule that will encompass the complexity of each and every case of assisted suicide, as the accounts in this book have gone some way to demonstrating. Life can be difficult, messy, fraught and unpredictable. What the law allowed Kay Gilderdale was for the facts to be presented to a panel of her equals: men and women capable of understanding something of the anguish and struggle the family went through and who could clearly appreciate that Kay, as she always had, acted to support her daughter.

If there was relief of sorts in Sussex because Kay Gilderdale had been acquitted, there was none at Frances Inglis's three-bedroom council home in the suburban sprawl of Dagenham.

This was the house where Thomas Inglis had grown up with his mother, lorry-driver father, elder brother Alex, and younger brother Michael. All three boys received a large part of their education there too, as Frances had taught them all at home at one stage or another.

This was the home from which young Tom would set off for a day's fishing, his favourite pastime, or to attend a local boxing club, or to be taken by his mother on outings to the Natural History or Science Museum.

But he was never to return there after his Saturday night out at the Ship & Anchor on 7 July 2007. That was the night when, as an innocent bystander to a fight, he was caught in the melee and hit from behind. The police urged him to get into an ambulance, which he did against his better judgement – Tom had always hated a fuss. These were the first steps towards his end, incidents that should have been no more than talking points.

Frances had thought about those moments hundreds of

times. Why, en route to a hospital did Tom fall from the moving ambulance?

Even at seven the next morning when the police called with the news of Tom's accident and she was driven to the hospital, it seemed that everything would be all right, that Tom would wake up and be himself again.

Seeing him in his drug-induced coma, however, had been a sign of what was to come. The operation she had not wanted to happen had pulled his skull open. Doctors had said that he had to have the operation; it was necessary or he could die, but what were they doing to him?

When her son opened his eyes, she sensed his emotion but could not sense Tom. He was unable to speak, he could not find her. They had all tried so hard. Sitting with him, talking to him, squeezing his hand. They tried to help him communicate, tried to show him how to blink once for yes or two for no, or squeeze hands, or anything at all. It never happened. Tom was gone.

He was allowed visitors only twice day and at set times. Frances was there, by his side in that hospital ward twice a day, every day, watching what was happening to her son. She knew how dreadful a fate this was for her once lively boy.

Tom had to be helped with his breathing, and every twenty minutes or so a nurse would have to remove his mucus with a small 'vacuum cleaner' appliance. Frances saw how much this terrified him, this noise every twenty minutes. Did it hinder his breathing while it was happening, she wondered? It must have been something because Tom – or the animal instinct that was buried in the shell of Tom – would panic. He would sweat and his muscles would go into spasms.

And to look at him broke every heart. Tom was being fed through a tube in his nose, there was a dip in his skull caused by the operation, and there was a gauge on his head measuring his cranial pressure. But the hardest thing of all to witness were the fits.

The brain damage was so severe that Tom was now an epileptic. Sometimes he would foam at the mouth, his arms and legs flailing, his body a torment beyond his control. The fits occurred two or three times a visit for the first few months – and then he barely moved at all. He had absolutely no control over movement; any movement was completely involuntary – except, perhaps, for his eye move-ments. He would scan the room with restless glances, occasionally letting his gaze rest on a face next to him.

What did he see? Fear, desolation, a void? How could his mother allow him such a painful existence . . . ?

In between her visits, Frances trawled the internet for information and support, but what she found and read there appalled her.

Alex said that his mother feared Tom would never recover despite being told by one doctor that there was a chance he might. He said of Frances, 'Of course she wanted to believe that he was getting better, we all wanted to believe that, but she really did want to know the truth.

'She knew how much Tom was suffering and I agree with her completely. If I had known that Tom did not have a chance I would have been on the same lines as her.

'She kept trying to make my dad see how bad Tom was. She was saying that she wanted people to agree with her that Tom wasn't getting better.

'A few days before the first attempt [on Tom's life] I said to my dad that I had a feeling that my mum was going to do something and he said that he had the same feeling.'

Tom's father spoke to one of the nurses at Queen's. Frances had said nothing directly, but for her a dangerous pressure to act was building. As Alex described it, 'Around that time, for a whole day, and I am not exaggerating it, she was constantly crying. She was quite "together" and when she was around Tom she would try not to be emotional; she would try and talk to him in an encouraging way and be happy around him.

'But she would sometimes walk out crying herself because she was having arguments with some of the nursing staff who were saying that Tom wasn't in pain when he obviously was.

'You could see when Tom's heartbeat went up and he started sweating and he looked uncomfortable and panicking. You could see his heart rate going up because he had a clip attached to him and you could see his oxygen levels and his heartbeat and blood pressure and things like that.'

Frances had lost a lot of weight. Everything in her life had narrowed to an absolute focus on her son and what was happening to him, locked inside his wrecked body.

Alex later revealed that his mother went to the hospital on three occasions with the intention of ending Tom's life and planned to take Max, the family's Labrador, with her to the hospital as there was a chance that Tom might be taken out into the fresh air in the hospital grounds and she could use the dog as a 'cover' to be outside.

On the first occasion, Frances had her family with her and on the second there were staff around. On the third, however, she carried out her first – and unsuccessful – attempt to end Tom's life by injecting him with heroin. She then left the hospital, assuming that he was dead.

Frances also assumed that when she went to the hospital the next day she would be arrested. However, on arriving there, she heard that they had resuscitated Tom.

'About two weeks after that, after they had done some tests at the hospital, the house was stormed by police,' Alex said. 'There was a knock on the door and there were loads of them, they were behind bushes and everything.

'I wasn't living with her [Frances] at the time but I was here just watching TV in the house. It was about seven p.m. They took her away that night and they searched the house and I was made to witness everything they did.'

Frances had been seen just before Tom had his cardiac arrest and she had been alone with him. She was now the prime suspect.

She denied it all to the police. She said in court later the reason that she denied everything was so that she would be left free to try again to help her son out of his misery. She had not been seeking to protect herself, but to buy more time.

But after her release, of course, she was not allowed any access to Tom at all. He then was moved – he had been moved before but this would be the last time – to the Neuro Centre at Sawbridgeworth.

Alex spoke about the strain that all the family were under: 'There were times when the family got all broke up by it all. There were times when my aunts Pat and Jane, Mum's sisters, weren't speaking to my mum, and there were times when I wasn't speaking to my mum or my dad wouldn't speak to her.'

Frances knew what she had to do next.

The staff started knocking on the door, and even though thirty minutes had passed, Frances was terrified that they would get in and resuscitate Tom. She could not fail him again.

Alex later said: 'The choices were, leave him and get on with her life, go about it the legal way and eventually starve him to death – it would have been in Tom's best interests but it would not have been fair on Tom to have put him through that – and there was the third option which is what she did, to release Tom in a painless way.

'It was not legal but who gives a shit about the law – it comes down to what is right and wrong. It does not matter what they say, the authorities. If it comes down to something as important as that and as morally right as that, it doesn't matter what laws some government says, you are not going to listen to them because it is the right thing to do.

'Look at what the Nazis did, that was legal because they made the laws. There are times when people need to ignore the law and just use your conscience. That is what my mother did.

'Almost all of the time the law is there for a reason and it is morally right, I am glad it is there. But technology changes, medicine changes, yet they leave the laws the same, they don't bother to redefine them.'

The family had to bear the loss not only of Tom, but now also of Frances. Alex recalled seeing his mother after her arrest: 'The first time we saw her after the arrest was when she was in court in the dock. It was a magistrate's court I think.

'She was crying because we had not been able to speak to her. We looked at her, and you know when you can say something even though you are not speaking at all, you get a message across with a look? And we were saying "it's all right, you did the right thing, Mum," and she was relieved that we weren't upset.'

Referring to people who want an assisted death, Alex said, 'There are two sets of people, those who can communicate and those who can't. They have an option for those who can't communicate and that is the removal of food and water. It has been going on for almost twenty years now. It's just the methods that they use, starving people to death. There is no need to do that. They could easily give people a peaceful way to die.

'We do have a system of euthanasia, the removal of food and water, but they don't want to say that because they torture some [people] to death and they don't want the responsibility.

'There is no need for it. If they could just change that method to a quick, painless way to die, then my mum would not be where she is now. It was being recommended to us. The end result is the same, death, but it is a much better way of doing it.

'The only reason that Tom would have gone through that long process is that the lawmakers are too cowardly to take any responsibility themselves. It's just because they can now stand back and say "we are not responsible" – all of them.

'She could easily have said in court that the balance of her mind was disturbed, but she did not want to do that.'

At the beginning of February 2010 Frances Inglis wrote as follows to the newspapers about her intention to appeal:

I want to make it clear that I am in no way opposed in principle to medical treatment and that if Tom could ever have recovered enough to enjoy any quality of life, I would have nursed him 24 hours a day for as long as necessary. But when there was no chance of any quality of life, I saw it as cruel and barbaric to allow – even force – him to suffer such agony.

I still live with the pain of the loss of my wonderful son and the awful knowledge of what he suffered, but I am comforted that he is no longer suffering and is at peace. What I did in releasing Tom was the most harrowing, the most heartbreaking and difficult thing I have ever had to do . . . I begged God for a miracle of recovery or Tom's peaceful death.

Frances's solicitor said the grounds of the appeal were that she believed the judge was wrong not to direct the jury to consider a defence known in law as 'slow burn provocation'. It applies to people who are driven to act when under extreme pressure, and is most commonly used in domestic violence cases where the victim retaliates after years of abuse.

As part of this approach it would be argued that Frances was driven to kill Tom after witnessing his suffering, and then learning that the only legal way to end his life would be to apply to the High Court for an order to withhold nutrition and hydration. Had the jury been allowed to consider that defence, they could have returned a verdict of manslaughter, which offers greater sentencing discretion, said lawyer Katie Wheatley, who also intended to appeal against Frances's sentence.

'The minimum term of nine years was far too long and failed to fully reflect the mitigating features of this case,' said Ms Wheatley.

After she was sentenced, Frances had said, 'Being in prison is nothing compared to what Tom was going through. If I had to face the death penalty to put him out of his suffering, I would still have done it. Parents should do anything for their children.

'I just am thankful to my family for supporting me. I was expecting to be convicted and I expected to go to prison. I knew what I was doing when I ended Tom's suffering. But this way, I've got a life sentence rather than Tom.'

Later, speaking from prison, she said: 'The whole thing has been like an earthquake in our lives. He was a wonderful son. He was happy and loving and kind. My life has never been the same since the accident. It was terrible during that period when I was not allowed to see him, knowing all that time that he was suffering.

'There may be people who say that it is better to have a son who is alive no matter how bad his condition than have a son who is dead. Well, those people are very selfish.

'I had no choice. I did the right thing. We are not talking about disability here, we are talking about someone who could not do anything for themselves at all. He was froth-ing at the mouth, biting his tongue and wagging his hand as though he was having a fit.

'He even broke his finger once in agitation. He needed twenty-four-hour care, he would not be able to come home from the hospital. If he could have spoken he would have asked me to do it. He was not able to say anything. They could have withheld treatment from him but that would be like killing him from thirst and hunger.

'If anyone says it was wrong of me to do it I would say to them that it would have been selfish to let him live. He did not want the quality of life that he had.'

And in a phrase that was fitting – not just in her case, but in all others where a mother has to make a decision of such magnitude for her child – Frances added one brief, emo-tional comment: 'I was not playing God.'

Epilogue

—

It is not too difficult to imagine that within the course of the next few years a British version of Dignitas might open its doors to those looking for 'an easeful death'.

No doubt such a move would be met with resistance, and the terms of such a clinic's business would come with a great many stipulations. But would that be such a terrible state of affairs? Clearly, a good many family members, caught up in the deteriorating health and wellbeing of a cherished loved one who repeatedly insists that they be allowed the right to end their life on their own terms, would be relieved that there existed such a route.

It would be a humane, professionally managed and pain-free exit that absolves relatives – parents, spouses, civil partners, adult children – or close friends – of physical involvement in that death, eases their emotional anguish as to how such a death can be staged as painlessly and smoothly as possible and, just as importantly, clarifies that, legally, they will not be guilty of any wrongdoing.

Such a route, a roll-back of the law as it stands, would have to overcome strong and vocal opposition. Even a discussion of the topic meets with controversy as the moral philosopher Baroness Warnock found when she wrote about the issue of euthanasia in 2008. Mary Warnock believes that those with dementia, those who see their lives as insufferable, those who believe their existence to be a drain on their families and the state, should be allowed to die.

But at what point can someone with dementia decide that their life is no longer worth living? And is it the case that euthanasia is the solution to the long-term care of those with degenerative disorders or those who, like Tom Inglis, are brain damaged? Is it not possible that a renewed commitment to research into prevention, treatment and cure of profoundly disabling conditions would be a more humane course of action?

Of course, even had a clinic built on the model of Dignitas already been in existence, it would not have helped Frances Inglis. The admission criteria are strict; the person who wishes to take their own life has to reiterate that intention several times to different medical and psychiatric professionals.

Such a clinic could, however, have helped Lynn Gilderdale. Once she had reached her conclusion in her struggle against ME, she would have been afforded the right to leave this life at a time of her choosing, her family at her side, and her mother free of the stress of administering the fatal drugs and the legal consequences of doing so.

The law is not perfect, and it is not possible to imagine that it ever will be. Yet as Baroness Finlay of Llandaff so concisely said of the law as it stands: 'It has a stern face and a kind heart.'

It was this kind heart that Kay Gilderdale found when the details of her case were heard in full by a panel of her peers.

Frances Inglis, however, did not escape the law's stern face, and neither had she really expected to, even before her last fateful trip to her son's bedside.

In October 2010, Frances' case was heard at the Court of Appeal. The judges were aware of the public interest in the case. They also accepted that 'mercy killing', euthanasia and assisted suicide are complex issues and that they are not just a matter for the courts. These are issues that should be addressed by Parliament, which in turn, should be 'reflective of the conscience of the nation'. But after that acknowledgement came a simple assertion: 'In this appeal we are constrained to apply the law as we find it to be. We cannot amend it, or ignore it'.

The law as it stands is unequivocal, as the Approved judgment issued by the Court stated, '… we must underline that the law of murder does not distinguish between murder committed for malevolent reasons and murder motivated by familial love.'

In the final analysis, the jury in the Inglis case and the Appeal Court judges were left with one incontrovertible fact: Tom did not speak. His mother spoke for him. The Appeal Court accepted that Frances was grief-stricken but also noted: 'She was convinced that she, and she alone, knew what was best for Thomas, to such an obsessive extent that any view to the contrary, however it was expressed, was to be rejected out of hand. This was not a moment or two of isolated thinking, but a settled intention'.

On this understanding, the conviction for murder stood. However, with such a difficult and sensitive case, the judges also stated: 'We must focus on all the critical facts and find a balance between them in which justice is appropriately tempered with mercy'. Perhaps this balance prompted their decision to reduce her minimum prison term to five years.

No one knew if Tom wanted to live or die. He did not end his life, it was taken. Perhaps Frances acted in a way that her son would have wished, but that could never be more than a stated belief. And on Thomas Inglis' silence and his mother's belief, the full weight of the law was brought to bear. It is a burden that Frances Inglis is willing to carry – and one that other mothers may find they are yet to endure.